THE TERMI
OF ANATOMY
AND PHYSIOLOGY

THE TERMINOLOGY OF ANATOMY AND PHYSIOLOGY

A PROGRAMMED APPROACH

Dale Pierre Layman, B.S., M.S., Ed.S.
Instructor
Department of Biology
Joliet Junior College
Joliet, Illinois

A WILEY MEDICAL PUBLICATION
JOHN WILEY & SONS
New York · Chichester · Brisbane · Toronto · Singapore

Library of Congress Cataloging in Publication Data:

Layman, Dale Pierre.
The terminology of anatomy and physiology.

(A Wiley medical publication)
1. Human physiology—Terminology—Programmed instruction. 2. Anatomy, Human—Terminology—Programmed instruction. I. Title. II. Series.
QP13.L39 1983 612′.0014 82-13448
ISBN 0-471-86262-2

Printed in the United States of America

10 9 8 7 6 5 4 3

PREFACE

This unique book focuses completely on the *terminology* of normal human anatomy and physiology. Written in a programmed format and intended for self-study, it constitutes a logical, integrated *system* for learning proper word spelling, interpretation, pronunciation, and usage.

The special "language" of human anatomy and physiology is based largely on Latin and Greek, two supposedly "dead" languages with which most modern college students are almost entirely unfamiliar! Is it any wonder, then, that so many people find the going difficult? They are suddenly confronted with the formidable task of learning a complex body of information about human form and function expressed in a strange technical language!

This book seeks to play a supplemental or helping role by providing the solid foundation upon which a sturdy house of word knowledge can be built. Rather than being forced to merely look up (and soon forget) an unfamiliar term, the student is shown how to *logically deduce* the meaning of the term by analysis and synthesis of its component word parts. In effect, the learner begins to see that the *terminology* of the body, like the body itself, can be better understood by dissecting it into its smaller parts and reassembling these parts in different combinations to yield an integrated whole.

Very little background knowledge is assumed. The programmed approach builds logically upon itself from the simple to the more complex. The technique has been very successful in the "sister" subject of medical terminology. The real beauty of this procedure is that the student becomes an *active participant* in the gradual, stepwise evolution of thorough competence in terminology.

Active learner involvement is promoted by

1. "Hinting" and "guiding" the student to make written responses in empty blanks within the text. Correctness of responses can be easily checked for immediate feedback.
2. Providing a *self-test* of individual roots, prefixes, and suffixes for each unit within the *appendix*.
3. Furnishing an alphabetized *index* citing the frames where the word parts and entire terms are introduced, permitting easy reference and review.

The program can be used either with or without a conventional anatomy/physiology textbook. Terms are segregated into the various body systems for study, but the sequence in which systems are learned can be altered to fit individual circumstances without loss of effectiveness.

Appropriate for introductory, college-level human anatomy and physiology, the book can also serve as a useful review for more advanced students in the life sciences. Perhaps even more important, it provides *new insight* into the subject matter, helping the learner to really "see" and appreciate the underlying meanings of terms otherwise memorized without much thought.

For example, the illustrations in this book, painstakingly prepared by Linda Cook DeVona, attempt to "bring out" in picture form many of the interesting verbal similes and analogies. The result, often highly colorful and amusing, helps to promote the general goal of understanding and retaining "mental pictures" of terms. When words have "personalities," they are very hard to forget!

Special thanks are extended to Robert F. Lee, College Representative for John Wiley & Sons, and to Andrea G. Stingelin, Editor of Nursing and Allied Health, for their interest, support, and good faith in the success of the project. Credit should also go to Jamee O'Brien and Sandy Kauzlaric for their student critique of the manuscript. Finally I would like to acknowledge the cooperation of my wife, Kathleen, and my son, Andrew, who had to live in the same house with me during the preparation of the book.

D.P.L.

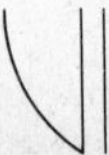

PRONUNCIATION KEY

The primary stress mark (′) is placed after the syllable bearing the heavier stress or accent; the secondary stress mark (') follows a syllable having a somewhat lighter stress, as in **com · men · da · tion** (kom'ən · dā′shən).

a	add, map	m	move, seem	u	up, done
ā	ace, rate	n	nice, tin	ûr	urn, term
air	care, air	ng	ring, song	yo͞o	use, few
a	palm, father	o	odd, hot	v	vain, eve
b	bat, rub	ō	open, so	w	win, away
ch	check, catch	ô	order, jaw	y	yet, yearn
d	dog, rod	oi	oil, boy	z	zest, muse
e	end, pet	ou	out, now	zh	vision, pleasure
ē	even, tree	o͞o	pool, food	ə	the schwa, an un-
f	fit, half	oo	took, full		stressed vowel
g	go, log	p	pit, stop		representing the
h	hope, hate	r	run, poor		sound spelled
i	it, give	s	see, pass		*a* in *above*
ī	ice, write	sh	sure, rush		*e* in *sicken*
j	joy, ledge	t	talk, sit		*i* in *clarity*
k	cool, take	th	thin, both		*o* in *melon*
l	look, rule	t͟h	this, bathe		*u* in *focus*

SOURCE: Slightly modified "Pronunciation Key" from *Funk & Wagnalls Standard College Dictionary*.

The schwa (ə) varies widely in quality from a sound close to the (u) in *up* to a sound close to the (i) in *it* as heard in pronunciations of such words as *ballot, custom, landed, horses*.

The (r) in final position as in *star* (stär) and before a consonant as in *heart* (härt) is regularly indicated in the respellings, but pronunciations without (r) are unquestionably reputable. Standard British is much like the speech of Eastern New England and the Lower South in this feature.

In a few words, such as *button* (but'n) and *sudden* (sud'n), no vowel appears in the unstressed syllable because the (n) constitutes the whole syllable.

CONTENTS

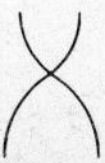

LIST OF TABLES

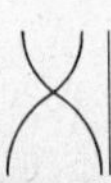

THE TERMINOLOGY OF ANATOMY AND PHYSIOLOGY

INTRODUCTION

Human anatomy and physiology as a discipline has been around for a long time. Through many centuries of thoughtful study an extensive technical vocabulary has gradually been developed to name, describe, and explain the varied aspects of body form and function.

This special "language" of anatomy and physiology is primarily based upon Latin and Greek word parts arranged in different patterns and sequences. To be a really effective learner in this field the student must be able to recognize, spell, pronounce, and utilize these word parts and their various combinations.

A *root* represents the main concept or "idea" of a word. In this book the roots are extracted directly from entire words. This simple procedure allows the learner to see directly how these roots can readily be combined with different *prefixes* and *suffixes*.

Prefixes are groups of letters or syllables that appear *before* the root. Prefixes can act like adjectives or adverbs to modify the idea of the root and thus make new word meanings.

Suffixes are groups of letters or syllables that come *after* the word root. Suffixes can act as adjectives, verbs, and even nouns in modifying the meaning of a word.

There are a limited number of commonly used prefixes and suffixes in human anatomy and physiology. The task is simply to learn these common word parts and then be able to recombine them with various roots to construct or analyze new terms.

The sequence is prefix—root—suffix. The *prefix* comes before or "leads into" the *root*, much like the *veins* come before or lead into the *heart*. And the *suffix* comes after or "leads out of" the *root*, just as the *arteries* come after or lead out of the *heart* (Fig. 1).

The next section, *How to Use This Book*, explains the exact procedure whereby active interaction with the text will help you to learn new terms.

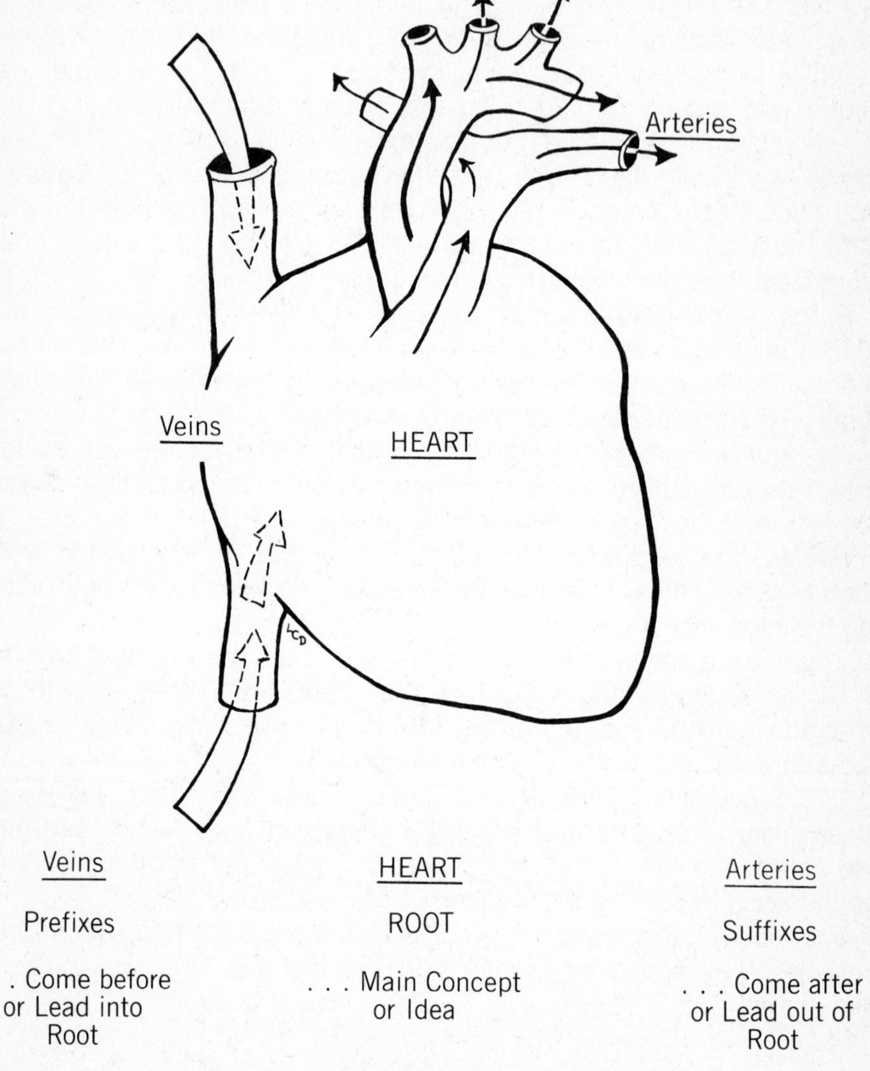

Figure 1. THE HEART AND WORD PARTS

HOW TO USE THIS BOOK

Directions: Take a folded piece of paper or cardboard. Use one that is long enough to cover up the answer column on the left side of the page.

1

This program is presented in terms of *learning frames*. A *learning frame* consists of a small package of information and an empty blank that you fill in. A single blank represents a response of just one word. A blank followed by an asterisk (*) calls for you to make a written answer of more than one word. Information provided within each frame, or information given in previous frames, is usually sufficient to enable you to fill in the blank correctly. Now, respond to the following statement: All the information below the number 1 is called a ______________.* Check to see if you filled in the correct answer by moving down your cover paper.

learning frame

2

Checking right away to see whether you have made the correct response gives your brain immediate feedback, speeding the learning process. This learning program consists of a number of learning frames, which offer you the advantage of immediate ______________. Check to see if you wrote in the correct answer by moving down your cover paper.

feedback

3

Right after filling in a blank always look immediately to discover whether you have written the appropriate answer. Use pencil rather than pen so you can keep things neat. Be sure to erase all mistakes and replace them with the correct responses. Organized, neat, and efficient learning with immediate feedback is called a learning ________.

program

4

When using this learning program remember not to peek ahead in a unit or skip over individual frames. Your brain is being presented with bits of new information in an orderly sequence that might be disrupted if you jump around. Work through each entire unit as a whole. Of course, you may look back at earlier learning frames for review. But remember, you are using a learning program in which new bits of information are being presented to you in an orderly ________.

sequence

5

Do not feel embarrassed or ashamed about making wrong answers. This is not a graded test but is rather a different way of learning. Much learning occurs by trial and error. You are expected to make some mistaken responses. Correct these mistakes immediately, and then reread the entire learning frame with the right answer filled in. You will learn immediately from your mistakes. After all, the brain learns much by ________.*

trial and error

6

Programmed learning is self-paced. By this is meant that you are free to learn the material at your own speed. It is not your speed, but rather your patience and persistence, in working through the program that is important. You are free to learn at your own ________.

pace (speed)

7

This program is *not* intended to replace a regular anatomy and physiology textbook or lab manual. It is designed to supplement or add to your learning experience. It will help you with the spelling, pronunciation, and proper use of the many technical terms you will encounter. Once you better understand the language of anatomy and physiology, the concepts presented in books, labs, and classroom will become clearer and easier to grasp. This learning program ______________ (adds to) your ability to understand "body language."

supplements

8

This learning program is *not* the same thing as a medical dictionary or a glossary. It is an organized *system* of learning and practicing with body terms, concepts, and phrases. It is largely based on the principle that actual doing and involvement is better than just passive textbook reading. Logical organized ______________ of programmed learning have been found very effective in helping students master difficult verbal material.

systems

9

To summarize, when you see a blank you should respond by writing in ______________ (one/more than one) word. And when you see a blank followed by an asterisk (*), you should respond by writing in ______________ (one/more than one) word.

one

more than one

10

It is fine to look back at earlier learning frames and refresh your memory of previous word parts. But you should not skip and peek ______________. You will remember to correct your mistakes ______________ (later/immediately).

ahead

immediately

11

This learning program is an organized logical

system (method)	____________ for presenting and reviewing verbal material, not a medical dictionary or word glossary.
language (terminology) Germany	**12** The subject of human anatomy and physiology, like any technical field, has its own particular language. Once you have learned anatomical and physiological ______________, you will be pleased to discover that learning essential body concepts is somewhat easier. The idea is simply to actively *work with* this terminology, like you would actively use the *German* language during a long visit to the country of ______________! After awhile you discover that the language comes more or less naturally to you! The terminology no longer seems quite so strange, foreboding, and confusing! The prevalent concepts and customs of the country become easier to understand. Welcome to the "country" of human anatomy and physiology! Good luck with the "language"!
	13 Before proceeding to the first unit be sure you look at the *Pronunciation Key* (p. vii) and become familiar with its symbols!

THE WORD-BUILDING SYSTEM: PREFIXES, ROOTS, AND SUFFIXES

---

root prefix suffix	**14** A ________ is the main concept or "idea" of a word. A ____________ comes *before* the main concept of a word and modifies word meaning. A ____________ comes *after* the main concept and likewise alters the total word meaning.
root suffix o	**15** In *speed/o/meter*, *speed* is the ________ or main idea, while *-meter* is the ____________. And the letter __ must represent a "combining vowel."
combining vowel	**16** The letter *o* is probably the most commonly used type of ________________________,* but *a*, *e*, *i*, and so forth, are often employed as well.
pelv; -meter	**17** In *pelv/i/meter* (pronounced pel vim′ ə tər) the root is ________, the suffix is ____________,

i	and the combining vowel is ___. There is no prefix present.
pelvimeter combining vowel	**18** You can see for yourself that it is easier to say *speedometer* than it is to say *speedmeter*, and that it is easier to say ______________ than to say *pelvmeter*. In each case a ______________________* has been placed between adjoining consonants in order to make word pronunciation easier and smoother.
crani; -meter o	**19** In *crani/o/meter* (krā nē om′ ə tər) the root is __________, the suffix is __________, and the combining vowel is the letter ___. No prefix is present.
Craniometer	**20** ______________________ is probably somewhat easier to pronounce than *cranimeter*, which lacks a combining vowel between the root and suffix. The general rule then is to use a combining vowel when connecting consonants of two different word parts, or when adding the combining vowel otherwise makes word pronunciation smoother, as between the *i* of *crani* and the *m* of *meter*.
-meter end	**21** Recall that in *speedometer*, *pelvimeter*, and *craniometer* the suffix in each case was ____________. You knew this simply by the placement of the word part at the ______ (beginning/end) of each of these three different terms.
	22 The suffix *-meter* actually means "an instrument used to measure (something)." The "something" is simply the root that precedes

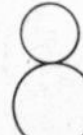

speedometer

-meter. For example a ________________ can be defined as "an instrument used to measure speed," such as the instrument on the dashboard of your car.

---

pelvimeter

23

Pelv comes from the Latin term for "bowl" or "basin." Build a term that means "an instrument used to measure a bowl": ____________ ____________.

---

craniometer

24

Crani derives from the Greek term for "skull." Build a term that means "an instrument used to measure the skull": ________________.

---

synthesize (construct, make)

25

Thus you see that you can both *analyze* or "break down" terms using slash marks (/) into their component word parts, and you can ________________ or "build up" new terms just from different combinations of separate word parts. These word parts always have the same meanings, but they can be arranged with many other word parts to make new terms. This is the essential idea of the terminology "system."

---

cephal/o/meter

cephal; o

-meter

26

For example, try to analyze *cephalometer* (sef ə lom ə tər) by rewriting the word and dividing it into a root, combining vowel, and suffix by inserting slash (/) marks: ____________ ____________. These marks help to indicate that ____________ is the root, __ is the combining vowel, and that ____________ is once again the suffix.

Cephal; pelv

27

Cephal comes from the Greek term for "head." ____________ ("head"), like ________ ("bowl")

crani

and ________ ("skull"), is an idea or root that can be combined with many different prefixes and suffixes to create new terms. In this book you will simply learn a set of roots involved with the anatomy and physiology of the different body systems, a list of common prefixes, and a list of suffixes. It is your skill in combining these separate word parts together to make new terms, and your ability to analyze terms you read into their component word parts, that will largely determine your competency in body "language."

28

The prefix *en-* means "inside of" or "within." So do *endo-* and *intra-*. *Encephal* means "____ ________________ ________________."* The *encephal* or "brain" does indeed lie "within the head"!

inside of or within the head

29

An ____/____________/__/__________ is "an instrument used to measure" the brain, which is located "inside of the head." The prefix in this term is ______. The prefix precedes the root.

en/cephal/o /meter (en sef ə lom′ ə tər)

en-

30

Examine Tables 1 and 2.

Table 1 "INSIDE OF" OR "WITHIN" PREFIXES

en-	in-
endo-	intra-

Table 2 "PERTAINING TO" SUFFIXES

-ac	-ary
-al	-ic
-alis	-ical
-an	-ine
-ar	-ous

31

Any of the prefixes and suffixes can be singly combined with a given root to make a new term. Using word parts from Tables 1 and 2, for instance, we can construct *intra/crani/al* (in tra krā' nē əl) and *crani/al* (krā'nē əl). The term ______________ is the one that contains no prefix.

cranial

32

______________ means "pertaining to the skull," while ______________ means "pertaining to (something) within the skull." In this case, ____________, not *en-*, is the prefix used to indicate location "inside of" or "within."

Cranial
intracranial
intra-

33

Both *cranial* and *intracranial* are alike in that they contain the root __________ and the suffix _____.

crani
-al

34

A high amount of ______________ pressure "within the skull" can lead to severe brain damage.

intracranial

35

Use the prefix *endo-*, the suffix *-ic*, and the root for "basin" to build a term meaning "referring to (something) within a basin": ________/________/____.

endo/pelv/ic
(en dō pel' vik)

36

The unborn baby has an ______________ location, being situated "within the bowl or basin" between the hip bones of its mother.

endopelvic

37

Observe that ______, the suffix in *endopelvic*, has the same meaning and use as ______, the suffix in *intracranial*. The choice of a partic-

-ic
-al

ular suffix from a group of suffixes having identical meaning is largely a matter of custom or usual convention for a particular root. The same can be said for prefixes having identical meanings. You will eventually learn that certain prefixes and suffixes just "sound better" with particular roots!

38

See Table 3.

Table 3 "OUTSIDE OF" AND "EXTERNAL" PREFIXES

ecto-
exo-
extra-

39

Ectopelvic (ek tō pel′ vik) means the exact opposite of ____________, while *extracranial* (eks trə krā′nē əl) has a meaning exactly opposite to ____________.

endopelvic

intracranial

40

An ____________ location is one "outside of the bowl," while an ____________ site refers to a place "outside of the skull." Thus both ________ and ________ are prefixes meaning "outside of."

ectopelvic

extracranial

ecto-

extra-

41

____________ pressure applied to the "external" surface of the "skull" must be very great in order to damage the soft brain within.

Extracranial

42

Now look at Table 4 to identify other prefixes indicating relative position or direction (page 13).

43

Using Table 4 and Table 2, rewrite *epicephalic*

Table 4 OTHER PREFIXES OF DIRECTION AND POSITION

ab-	"away from"	*hypo-*	"below; deficient"
ad-	"toward"	*inter-*	"between"
af-	"toward"	*met-, meta-*	"after"
ana-	"up; toward; apart"	*par-, para-*	"beside"
anti-	"against"	*peri-*	"around"
de-	"away from"	*pro-*	"before; first"
dia-	"through"	*sub-*	"below; beneath; under"
ef-	"out of; away from"	*trans-*	"across"
epi-	"upon"	*tel-, telo-*	"end"
ex-	"out of; away from"		

epi/cephal/ic

(ep i sə fal′ ik) and insert slash marks (/) to divide it into its prefix, root, and suffix: ______ ______________.

Epi-
epicephalic

44
________ means "upon." A hat is generally placed into an ________________ ("upon the head") position.

45
See Table 5 for prefixes involving numbers and relative proportions.

Table 5 PREFIXES OF NUMBER AND PROPORTION

bi-	"double; two; twice"	*pan-*	"all"
di-	"double; two; twice"	*poly-*	"many"
hyper-	"above normal; excessive"	*quadri-*	"four"
iso-	"same; equal"	*semi-*	"partial; partially; half"
mono-	"single"	*tri-*	"three"

46
Using Table 5 and Table 2, rewrite *dipelvic* (dī pel′ vik) and insert slash marks (/) to subdivide

di/pelv/ic di-; pelv- -ic	it into its component parts: ______________. The prefix is ______, the root is __________, and the suffix is ______. No combining vowel is present.
dipelvic	**47** A ________________ female would be one that literally had "two bowls"!
	48 Review Table 6 for various miscellaneous prefixes.

Table 6 MISCELLANEOUS PREFIXES

a-	"not; without"	*neo-*	"new"
auto-	"self"	*re-*	"back; again"
in-	"not"	*syn-*	"together"

neo/crani/al neo- crani -al	**49** Using Table 6 and Table 2, rewrite *neocranial* (nē ō krā′ nē əl) and subdivide it with slash marks into its component word parts: ______________________. The prefix is ________, the root is __________, and the suffix is ______.
neocranial	**50** The ____________________ ("pertaining to new skull") tissue, at first soft and pliable, later becomes rock-hard.
adjectives	**51** So far you have been building and analyzing terms using several roots and a number of different types of prefixes. But only one group of suffixes, the "pertaining to" (Table 2) suffixes, have been used. Such suffixes as *-ic* and *-al*, when placed on the ends of words, make the words ________________ (nouns/adjectives/verbs) that modify the meaning of other words. Another group of suffixes, the "presence of"

suffixes, make terms into nouns that can stand alone. These suffixes are listed in Table 7.

Table 7 "PRESENCE OF" SUFFIXES

-a	-on
-e	-um
-is	-us

52

Using Tables 4 and 7, subdivide *telencephalon* (tel en sef′ ə lon) by means of slash marks: ______________. Here the prefix is not *en-* but rather ________, because it is the word part that comes first. *En-* is included with *cephal* to make the single root, ____________ ("within head" or "brain"). The suffix is ______.

tel/encephal/on

tel-

encephal

-on

53

______________ literally means "presence of the end-brain." The suffix ______ means "presence of," and the prefix ________ means "end."

Telencephalon

-on

tel-

54

The ______________ is the "end" of the "brain present" in the front, and it is responsible for most of our conscious thought.

telencephalon

55

Various miscellaneous suffixes are described in Table 8 (page 16).

56

Use Table 8 to help you construct a term meaning "the study of bowls": ____________. To do this you must employ the suffix ____________.

pelvology

-ology

Table 8 MISCELLANEOUS SUFFIXES

Suffix	Meaning
-able	"able"
-ary	"characterized by"
-ase	"splitter"
-ate	"something which"
-elle	"tiny; miniature"
-ens	"one that"
-ent	"one that"
-er	"a thing that"
-form	"form; like"
-gen	"produce"
-id	"belonging to a group"
-ide	"a compound with two different parts"
-il	"tiny; little; small"
-in	"a neutral substance"
-ine	"a basic substance
-ion	"the act or process of"
-ity	"condition of being"
-le	"tiny"
-mere	"segment"
-oid	"resembling; steroid"
-ois	"resembling"
-ol	"alcohol; related to alcohol"
-ole	"tiny"
-ology	"the study of"
-or	"one that; one who"
-ory	"characterized by"
-ose	"a type of sugar or other carbohydrate"
-osis	"condition of"
-poiesis	"formation of"
-stasis	"control of"
-sterone	"steroid"
-tion	"the act or process of"
-ule	"tiny"
-y	"action, process, or condition of"

57

Subdivide *pelvology* (pel vol′ ə jē) with slashes: ____________. The root in this term is ______.

pelv/ology

pelv

58

____________ involves the study of the bony basin between the hip bones. This bony basin is called the *pelvis* (pel′ vis).

Pelvology

59

Employing Table 7, you can literally define *pelvis* as "____________."* Here the suffix ______ means "presence of."

presence of a basin (bowl)

-is

Answers	Frames
Pelvology pelvimeter	**60** ________ or "study of" the bony "pelvis" is conducted with the aid of a ________ ("instrument used to measure the pelvis").
crani/ology (krā nē ol′ ə jē)	**61** Now *you* build ________/________, a term for "study of the skull."
pelv; cephal crani	**62** Isn't this fun? Can you see that the possibilities for creating new terms are almost endless? All you need to do is combine a given root with certain prefixes and suffixes! For example, every body term discussed in this section involved only one of three different roots: ________ ("bowl"), ________ ("head"), and ________ ("skull").
system (method, process, etc.)	**63** In succeeding units you will see the prefixes and suffixes of this section again, and you will learn how they combine with various roots of the different body systems. At the beginning of each new section you will see a list of terms. These are the terms that you will use to fill in the provided blanks. By practice and logical thinking you will make your way, step by step, through the anatomy and physiology of the word-building ________.
	64 Now begin your study with Unit 1. (*Note*: You may want to rework this section on word-building one or two more times first! Be sure you have a basic idea of what the terminology system is all about!)

UNIT 1

INTRODUCTION TO TERMS OF STRUCTURE AND FUNCTION

65
The study of the human body is subdivided into two major areas: body structure and body function. *Anatomy* (pronounced ə nat′ ə mē) is the science of body structure.

---

anatomy

66
Terminology, the study of words and their component parts, like the human body itself, has an ______________ (science of structure).

---

gross

67
Both in terminology and in anatomy it is often desirable to break down the whole into its component parts, or to build a greater structure by properly assembling smaller parts. In each case our understanding increases when we can see the "big picture" of how things fit together. *Gross* (pronounced grōs) means "big" or "large." Large body structures are studied in the science of __________ anatomy. Here "large" means that the structures are visible to the naked eye.

Gross

68
__________ (large) anatomy has traditionally involved the dissection or "cutting up" of bodies in order to study their inner structure.

Table 1.1 TERMS OF GENERAL BODY STRUCTURE

abdomen	external	plane
abdominal	gross	posterior
abdominopelvic	hypochondriac	proximal
anatomic	hypogastric	sagittal
anatomical	iliac	section
anatomy	ilium	superior
anterior	inferior	suture
buccal	internal	thoracic
caudal	lateral	thorax
cephalic	lumbar	transverse
coronal	medial	umbilical
cranial	mesial	umbilicus
diaphragm	oral	ventral
distal	parietal	vertebral
dorsal	pelvic	viscera
epigastric	pelvis	visceral

69

Just as the body can be subdivided with knives or scalpels to analyze its component parts, so can a body term often be subdivided by slash marks into its individual word parts. For example we can "cut up" *anatomy* in this fashion, where *tom*, the ________ (main concept) means "cut."

root

70

The prefix in *anatomy* must be ________, because it precedes the root *tom*. Likewise the suffix in *anatomy* must be ____, because it immediately follows *tom* (Fig. 1.1).

ana-

-y

71

Recall from Table 4 (frame 42) that ________ is a prefix meaning "up; toward; apart." And Table 8 (frame 55) lists ____ as a suffix for "action, process, or condition." The literal or exact meaning of ____________ is thus "the process of cutting up." What an appropri-

ana-

-y

anatomy

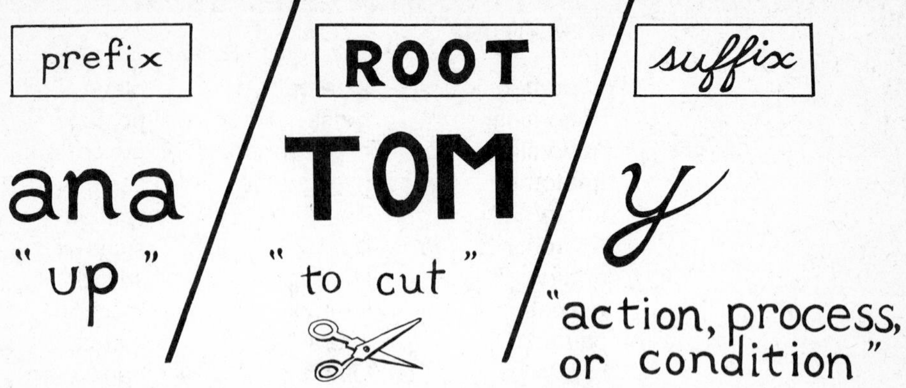

Figure 1.1. DISSECTION OF "ANATOMY"

Answers	Frame
	ate and logical name for this "cutting" science that analyzes body structure!
the process of before suffix	**72** Note in frame 71 that "the process of" part of the English translation of the suffix *-y*, comes ________ (before/after) the English translation of the root and prefix. This example illustrates the general rule that most of the time, the *last* part or ____________ (prefix/suffix) of a term comes *first* in the English definition of the term!
ana/tom/ic ana/tom/ical	**73** Take the terms *anatomic* (an ə tom′ ik) and *anatomical* (an ə tom′ i kəl). *Anatomic* is subdivided with slash marks as ____________________, while *anatomical* is properly subdivided as ________________________.
-ic -ical 2	**74** The suffix in *anatomic* is ______, while the suffix in *anatomical* is __________. How do we know this? We look for the appropriate suffixes in our tables of suffixes provided in the *Word-Building* section. We find both *-ic* and *-ical* listed in Table __ (frame 30).

75
The suffixes *-ical* and *-ic* mean "______________________________________." Thus both *anatomical* and *anatomic* are translated as "____." Note that the "pertaining to" portion, representing a suffix, comes first in the English translation of these terms. This illustrates the general rule mentioned earlier.

pertaining to
pertaining to
cutting up

76
The ________________________ position is the blueprint or reference used to describe the relative locations of different body structures. It serves as a standard "road map" to direct the "cutting up" of the body.

anatomic
(anatomical)

77
To see deep *internal* structures hidden beneath the skin we must "cut up" the body. *Intern* is a root meaning "inside of." Subdivide *internal* with slash marks: __________________________.

intern/al
(in tûr′ nəl)

78
Extern is a root meaning "outside of." Build a term that means the exact opposite of *internal*: ________________________.

external
(eks tûr′ nəl)

79
The suffix in both *internal* and *external* is _______, the same one used in *cranial* (frame 33). This suffix means "__________________________________." (See Table 2, frame 30, if in doubt.)

-al
pertaining to

80
Whereas *internal* means "pertaining to the inside of (something)," *external* means "____."

pertaining to
the outside of
(something)

81

The suffix, *-al*, always means "________________________," regardless of what particular root it happens to follow. This built-in redundancy of meaning is the real beauty of the terminology system!

pertaining to (referring to)

82

Examine *visceral* (vis' ər əl) and *parietal* (pə rī' ə təl). You should immediately note that each term contains the suffix ______; that is, they both "refer to" something.

-al

83

Viscer is a root for "internal organs," while *pariet* means "wall." Therefore ____________/____ is a term "referring to the internal organs" within some body cavity; and ____________/____ is a term "referring to the wall" of that body cavity.

viscer/al

pariet/al

84

Parietal and *visceral* are often used to describe relative position or direction within some body cavity. For instance, if we cut toward the internal organs located deep within a body cavity, we are moving in a ______________ ("referring to the internal organs") direction.

visceral

85

The internal organs are technically called the *viscera* (vis' ər ə). If something in a cavity is closer to the wall than it is to the ____________ ("internal organs") in the middle of the cavity, we say that it is ______________ ("pertaining to the wall") (Fig. 1.2).

viscera

parietal

86

Parietal is to ______________ as *external* is to ______________; that is, they pertain to opposite directions!

visceral

internal

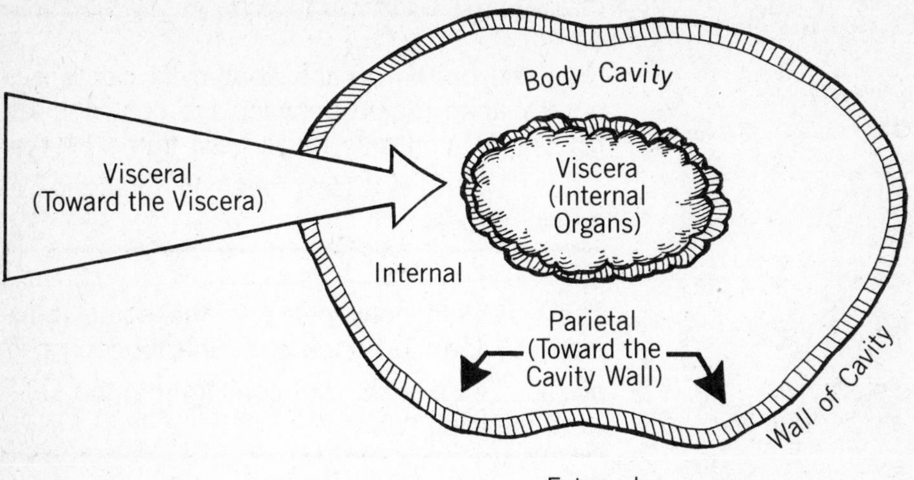

Figure 1.2. CROSS-SECTION THROUGH BODY TRUNK

Answer	Frame
visceral	**87** The stomach is ________ (parietal/visceral) to the wall of the cavity that contains it.
-al	**88** The stomach lies within the *abdominal* (ab dom′ i nəl) cavity. The root in *abdominal* is *abdomin*, while the suffix once again is ____.
Abdomin/al	**89** *Abdomin* represents the *abdomen* (ab dō′ mən, ab′ də mən). The abdomen is the middle section of the body trunk. ________/____ means "referring or pertaining to the abdomen (trunk midsection)."
viscera abdominal parietal	**90** The stomach and other nearby ________ ("internal organs") are found within the ________ ("trunk midsection") cavity. Consequently, the wall of this cavity is ________ (parietal/visceral) to the organs lying within.

Answer	Frame
pelvis	**91** Near the bottom of the abdominal cavity is a bowl-shaped region between the right and left hip bones. You may recall from frame 59 that ____________ is a term meaning "presence of a bowl or basin."
Pelv	**92** The so-called bony pelvis is the actual bowl made by the hip bones and other bones nearby. ________ is the root coming from the Latin word meaning "bowl."
pelvic -ic	**93** The ____________ ("bowl") *cavity* is the hollow space within the bony pelvis. Recall from frame 46 that ______, not *-al*, is the "pertaining to" suffix usually placed after *pelv*.
o abdominopelvic (ab dom′ i nō pel′ vik)	**94** You might also remember from the *Word-Building* section that __ is probably the most common combining vowel. Now *you* try to create a term that means "referring to the trunk midsection and the bowl": ________________ ________________.
abdomin/o/pelv/ic abdomin; pelv	**95** Analyze *abdominopelvic* by inserting slashes: ______________________________ _____. Observe that this term contains two different roots, ______________ and ________, attached together by a combining vowel.
Abdominopelvic	**96** A term with more than one root is called a *compound word*. ____________________ _____ is thus a compound word.
	97 There is no actual physical separation between the abdominal and pelvic cavities. They are

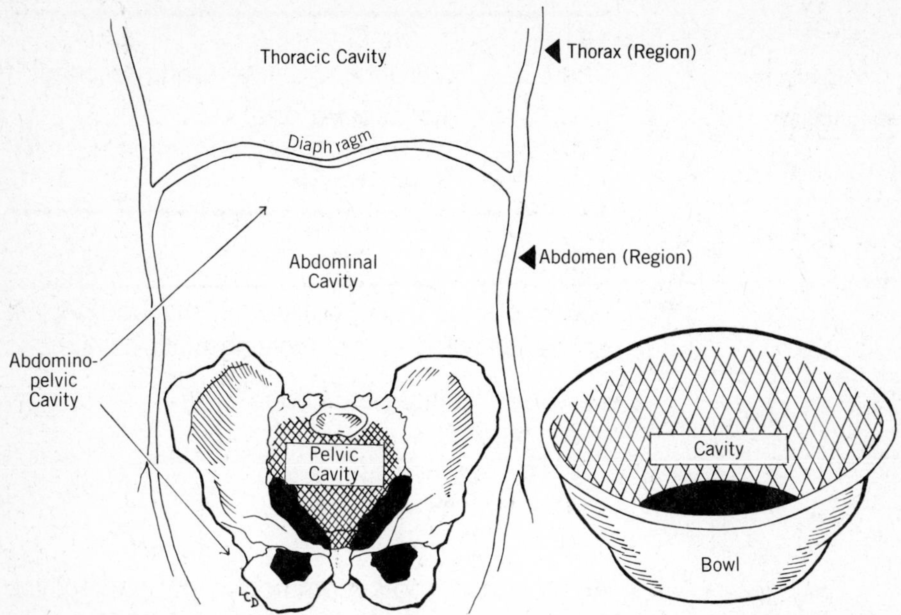

Figure 1.3. RELATIONSHIPS OF ABDOMINAL AND THORACIC CAVITIES

abdominopelvic	both just one big ______________ cavity (Fig. 1.3).
diaphragm (dī′ ə fram)	**98** Examine Figure 1.3. Which term do you think comes from the Greek for "partition or barrier"? Write it here: ______________.
diaphragm	**99** The ______________ is the "barrier" muscle that separates the *thoracic* (thō ras′ ik) from the abdominopelvic cavity.
thorac	**100** Since *thoracic* means "pertaining to the chest" then ______________ must be the root for "chest." The *thorax* (thō′ raks) is the actual term used for the chest. But the final *x* is always changed to *c* before making any other term involving the chest.

thorac/ic

diaphragm

101
The ______/___ ("referring to chest") *cavity* lies just above the ________ ("partition"), whereas the *abdominopelvic cavity* lies immediately below.

thorax

102
The cavity within the ________ ("chest") is just one of many cavities in the body. Look at the following roots involving body cavities:

vertebr "jointed backbone"
or "mouth"
bucc "cheek"
dors "back"
ventr "belly"

All of these roots commonly form adjectives with *-al*.

vertebr/al (vər′ tə brəl)

dors/al (dôr′ səl)

103
The ______/___ *canal* is the hollow space lying within the "jointed backbone" or spine. This space is part of the _____/___ *cavity* in the "back."

oral; buccal (ôr′ əl, ō′ rəl; buk′ əl)

ventr/al (ven′ trəl)

104
The _____ ("mouth") or ______ ("cheek") *cavity* lies above the _____/___ *cavity* located in the front or "belly" region of the body.

bucc/al

or/al

-al

105
Buccal is subdivided as _____/___, and *oral* as ___/___. In each case the suffix is ____.

vertebral

cranial

dorsal

106
Both the __________ ("pertaining to jointed backbones") *canal* and the __________ ("referring to the skull," frame 32) *cavity* lie within the ________ ("back") *cavity*. We can often use *-al* as a suffix with

dors	______, the root for "back," when we want to employ "back" as an adjective modifying some other word.
thoracic abdominopelvic ventral -ic -al	**107** Both the ______ ("chest") cavity and the ______ ("trunk midsection and bowl") cavity are usually included within the so-called ______ ("belly") cavity in the front of the body. It is customary to use the suffix ______ with *thorac* and the suffix ______ with *ventr*.
gross	**108** Besides study of the body cavities, ______ ("large") anatomy involves the use of *planes* or imaginary flat sheets to artificially separate body regions from one another.
planes abdomen	**109** For example, ______ (imaginary flat sheets) can be passed in both horizontal and vertical directions through the ______ ("trunk midsection"), dividing it into nine different regions (Fig. 1.4).
	110 Examination of Figure 1.4 reveals that these abdominal regions are sequentially numbered. The names of these regions include the following set of roots: *chondr* "cartilage; gristle" *gastr* "stomach" *lumb* "loins" *ili* "flank" *umbilic* "pit"
hypo/chondr/i/ac	**111** Again look at Figure 1.4. Use slashes to subdivide *hypochondriac* (hī pō kon′ drē ak): ______, *hypogastric*

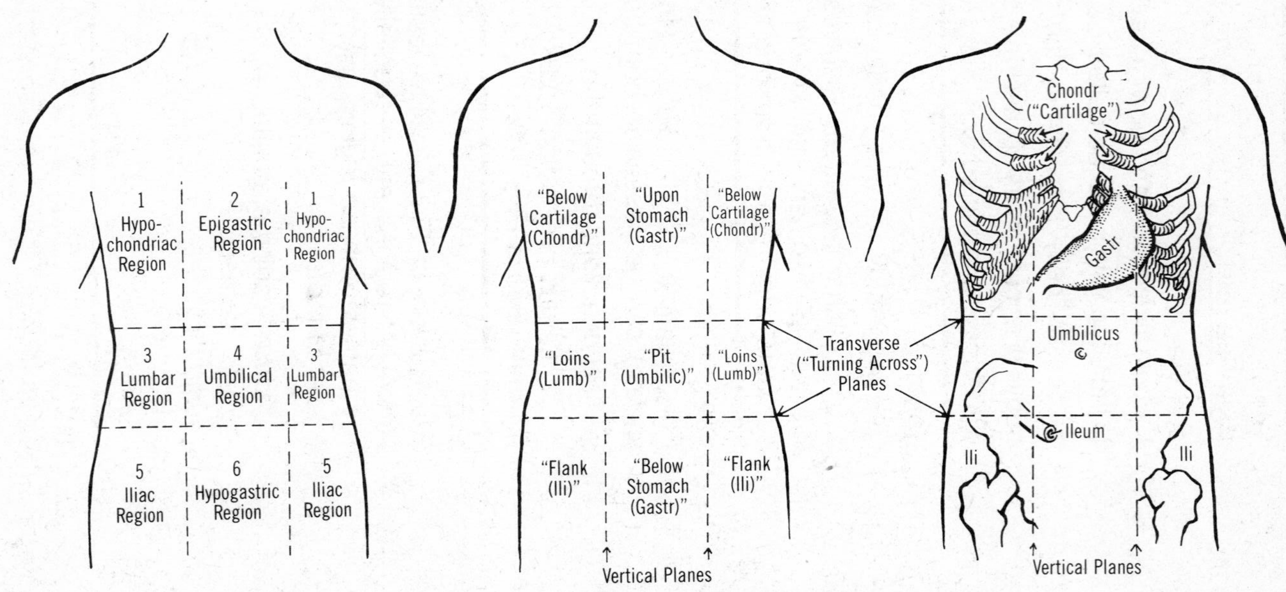

Figure 1.4. ABDOMINAL REGIONS

hypo/gastr/ic epi/gastr/ic lumb/ar umbilic/al ili/ac	(hī pō gas′ trik): ______________ ___, *epigastric* (ep i gas′ trik): ______________ ______________, *lumbar* (lum′ bär, lum′ bər): ___ ______________, *umbilical* (um bil′ i kəl): ___ ______________, and *iliac* (il ē ak): ___ ______.
prefix suffix	**112** Did you divide all the terms in frame 111 correctly? The general procedure is to isolate the roots, which you were given, with slash marks. Anything preceding these roots must then be a ______________, and anything following them must be a ______________, with the possible addition of a combining vowel in between.
-ac; -ic -ar; -al	**113** The four different suffixes found within the terms of frame 111 are: ______, ______, ______, and ______, all of them meaning "pertaining to." (Consult Table 2, frame 30, for confirmation.) The matter of which particular "pertaining to" suffix goes with each different root is simply a matter of usual custom or common practice.
hypo- hypochondriac hypogastric	**114** Two of the terms in frame 111 contain the prefix __________, which means "below." (Review Table 4, frame 42). These terms are ______________ ("referring to the area below cartilage") and ______________ ("referring to the area below the stomach").
hypogastric	**115** By examining Figure 1.4 again you will observe that the ______________ *region*, number (6) on the diagram, does indeed lie "below the stomach," which is located mostly

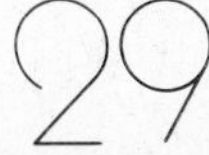

Gastr	within region (2). ________ is the root for "stomach."
Chondr hypochondriac i	**116** ________ means "cartilage" or "gristle," the hard rubbery material found at the ends of many bones. Much of the *right* and *left* ________ *regions* of the abdomen (Fig. 1.4) do indeed lie "below the cartilage" that tips the front ends of the upper ribs! The letter __ is the combining vowel in this term.
epigastric epi-	**117** One term listed in frame 111, ________, includes ________, a prefix for "upon." (Consult Table 4, frame 42, for help.)
epigastric	**118** The upper portion of the ________ *region* (Fig. 1.4) lies "upon the stomach," which is located in the lower portion. The suffix *-ic* is employed in this term.
umbilical umbilic	**119** The name of region (4) in Figure 1.4 is the ________ ("pertaining to the pit") *region*, where *ic* is part of the root, ________. The suffix in this case is *-al* ("pertaining to").
presence of umbilic/us (um bil′ i kəs)	**120** The suffix, *-us*, means "________."* (Review Table 7, frame 51.) Use this suffix to build ________/____, a term meaning "presence of a pit."
umbilicus	**121** The ________ is commonly called the "navel" or "belly-button." It represents the small "pit present" in the middle of the abdo-

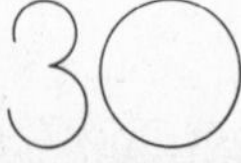

umbilical	men where the ______________ ("pertaining to the pit") *cord* attached the unborn child to a special organ in the mother's womb.
umbilical	**122** Return to Figure 1.4. On each side of the ______________ ("referring to the navel") region we have the *lumbar* regions of the abdomen.
lumb/ar lumb -ar	**123** Subdivide *lumbar*: ____________. The root in *lumbar* is _______, while the suffix is _____. Some terms, like *lumbar*, have no prefix.
loins referring to the loins (small of back)	**124** According to frame 110 the meaning of *lumb* is "_________," or the small of the back. Then *lumbar* is used as an adjective that means "______________________________ ____."*
lumbar	**125** A spinal tap is often called a __________ puncture because a hollow needle is inserted into the "small of the back" in order to withdraw spinal fluid.
ili ili -ac	**126** According to frame 110 _____ is the root for "flank." The root in *iliac* is _____, and the suffix is _____.
iliac	**127** The __________ ("pertaining to flank") region is near the hips (Fig. 1.4).
ili/um -um	**128** Analyze *ilium* (il′ ē əm) with slashes: _____/____. The suffix in *ilium* is _____. This suffix has the same meaning as *-us* in *umbilicus*.

presence of the flank -um	**129** *Ilium* means "________________________________ ____________,"* because ______ means "presence of."
ilium iliac	**130** The __________ forms the "flank" and represents the wide upper area of each hip bone. See if you can feel your own __________ *crest* or upper hip ridge by pressing your fingertips into the sides of your "flanks."
transverse trans- presence of	**131** Take one last look at Figure 1.4. Observe that two horizontal or __________________ *planes* have been passed across the abdomen. Table 4 (frame 42) lists __________ as a prefix for "across." *Vers* is a root meaning "turn." And according to Table 7 (frame 51) *-e* is a suffix for "________________ ____."*
trans/vers/e	**132** Thus __________/________/__ means "presence of a turning across."
the act or process of sect/ion	**133** *Sect* is a root for "cut," while Table 8 (frame 55) relates that *-ion* is a suffix for "______ ________________________________."* Thus a ________/______ results from "the act or process of cutting" the body. It is an actual physical cut made through some body plane.
transverse	**134** A ____________________ *section* is one made by a knife "turning across" the body in a left-right horizontal manner. This so-called *cross section* divides the body into upper and lower portions, identified with terms like

superior
cranial
cephalic (sə fal′ ik)
inferior
caudal (kô′ dəl)

---

cephal
crani
Crani/al

135
Recall from frame 27 that ______ is the root for "head" and that ______ is the root for "skull." ______/____(frame 32) "refers to the skull."

---

cephal/ic

136
What must we do to *epicephalic* (frame 43) to create ______/____, a term "pertaining to the head"?

---

caud/al

137
If *caud* means "tail" in Latin then ______/____ "refers to" a direction toward the foot or "tail" end of the body.

Cephalic
cranial
transverse

138
______, an adjective indicating the "head" end of the body, and ______, an adjective denoting the end of the body with the "skull," are used in the same way to indicate position *above* some imaginary ______ ______(horizontal) *plane*.

---

caudal

139
The ______ or "tail" end of the body indicates location *below* some transverse plane.

---

cephalic
cranial
caudal

140
Practicing with the terms presented in frames 138–139 we can say that the chin is ______ ______ or ______ to the chest, and that the chest is ______ to the chin. In our imagination we have passed a transverse

	plane through the neck, separating the chin above at the "head" or "skull" end from the chest below at the "tail" end of the body.
infer/i/or infer -or i	**141** If *superior* is subdivided as *super/i/or*, then *inferior* is probably subdivided as ______________, where __________ is the root and ______ is the suffix. In this case the letter __ serves as the combining vowel.
one that one who	**142** The suffix *-or* is found in Table 8 (frame 55). It means "________________"* or "______________."*
below; superior inferior	**143** The roots *super* and *infer* are opposites. That is, if *super* means "above" then *infer* means "________________;" and ________________ means "one that is above," while ________________ means "one that is below."
superior	**144** If a body part is *inferior* to some other body part then it is "below" it. Conversely, if a body part is ________________ to some other body part then it is "above" the part in question.
superior	**145** The chin is *cephalic, cranial*, or ________________ to the chest. These three adjectives all indicate a relative position "above" something else.
inferior	**146** The chest is *caudal* or ________________ to the chin. These two adjectives indicate relative position "below" something else.

Answers	Frame
sutur/e (syoo′ chər, soo′ chər) seam	**147** If *sutur* is a root for "seam" then ________/__ is "presence of a seam," where the suffix is the same as that in *transverse* (frame 132). This is actually a joint which forms a thin crack holding the bones of the face and skull together like a "________" uniting the separate patches of a bed quilt.
sagitt/al (saj′ i təl)	**148** *Sagitt* is Latin for "arrow." Using the suffix found in *caudal* (frame 137), build a term that means "referring to an arrow": ________/____.
coron/al (kôr′ ə nəl, kə rō′ nəl)	**149** *Coron* means "crown." Use the suffix in *cranial* (frame 135) to construct ________/____, a term "pertaining to a crown."
Sagittal suture	**150** ____________________* "refers to" the "presence of" a crack or "seam" that would be created by an "arrow" passing back to front over the middle of the top of the skull (Fig. 1.5).
Coronal suture	**151** ____________________* "refers to" the "presence of" a crack or "seam" passing left to right across the front of the top of the skull, forming a pattern much like the "crown" on a prince's head (Fig. 1.5).
sagittal middle	**152** A plane can be guided right down through the middle of the ____________("arrow") *suture*, dividing the body into exactly equal left and right halves. This plane is often called the "midsagittal plane" or "body midline." *Mid-* obviously means "__________."

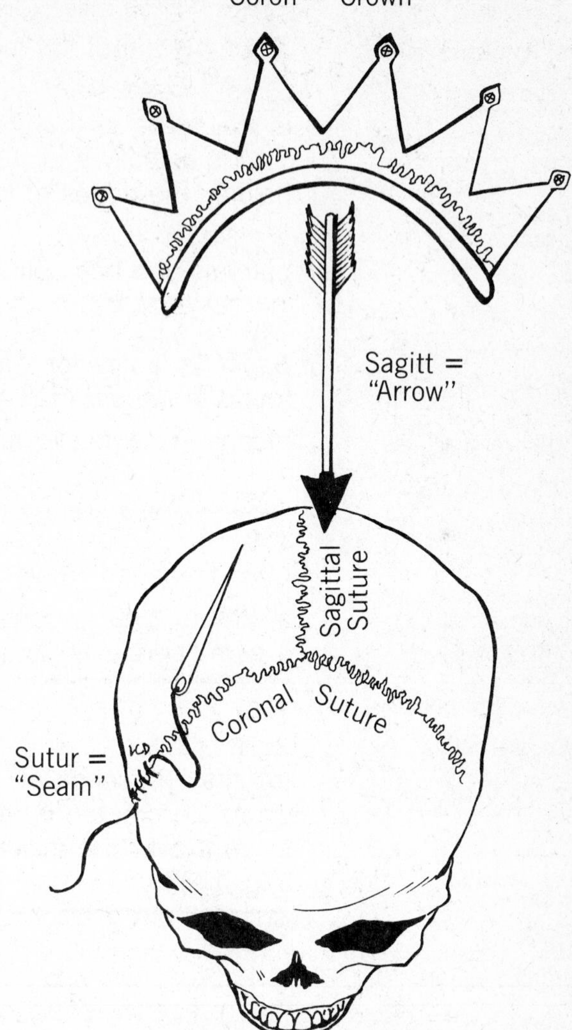

Figure 1.5. SKULL—SUPERIOR ASPECT

153
Look at the following roots:

medi "middle"
mes "middle"
later "side"

154
Employ the suffix in *coronal* (frame 149) to build two different terms "pertaining to

medi/al (mē′ dē əl) mes/i/al (mē′ zē əl)	the middle": ________/____ and ______/__/____.
medial mesial	**155** The term __________ sounds just fine. But combining vowel *i* must be added to *mes* to yield __________, a term that would otherwise sound too much like the disease called *measles*!
medial; mesial	**156** The nose is __________ or __________ to the eyes. By this is meant that the nose is closer to the body midline (*midsagittal plane*) than are the eyes.
later/al (lat′ ər əl) opposite	**157** Apply the suffix in *buccal* (frame 105) to make a term "referring to the side": __________/____. This term is __________(similar/opposite) in meaning to *medial*.
lateral	**158** The eyes are __________ to the nose. In other words the eyes are "to the side of" the nose, farther from the *body midline*.
coronal	**159** A *frontal* or __________("crown") plane divides the body into front and back portions, allowing us to distinguish structures from each other.
anter/i/or (an tir′ ē ər) poster/i/or (pos tir′ ē ər)	**160** Given *anter/i* "front" and *poster/i* "behind," use the suffix found within *super/i/or* to build two terms, the first meaning "one that is in front," and the second meaning "one that is behind or in the rear": __________/__/____ and __________/__/____.
anterior	**161** You can probably guess that __________

ventral	______ (anterior/posterior) is used interchangeably with ______________ ("pertaining to the belly," frame 104) in humans.
Posterior dorsal	**162** __________________ (the opposite of *anterior*) is often used interchangeably with ______ ("referring to the back," frame 103) in humans. Walking upright on two legs, the human has a "belly" in the "front" while the "back" follows "behind" or "in the rear."
anterior posterior dorsal	**163** The nose is ______________ ("in front of") or *ventral* to the forehead, but the forehead is __________________ ("in the rear of") or ____________ to ("in back of") the nose.
-al	**164** Finally, two terms are often used to indicate relative closeness of body parts to the shoulder or to the hip. These terms are *proximal* (prok′ si məl) and *distal* (dis′ təl). You can probably guess that the suffix in each case is ______ ("pertaining to").
dist proxim	**165** In frame 164 ________ is the root for far "distance," whereas ____________ is the root for "near" or "close proximity."
proximal distal	**166** A ________________ structure lies "near" the origin (hip or shoulder) of a body limb, whereas a ____________ structure lies some "distance" away.
proximal distal	**167** For example, the knee is ________________ to the ankle, but the ankle is ____________ to the knee.

distal proximal	**168** The wrist is ________ to the elbow, but the elbow is ________ to the wrist.

Table 1.2 TERMS OF GENERAL BODY FUNCTION

homeostasis	physiological
physiologic	physiology

anatomy	**169** Just as ________ ("the process of cutting up") involves determination of the shape, size, and composition of body parts, *physiology* (fiz ē ol′ ə jē) involves body functions.
	170 Look at: *physiology* *physiologic* (fiz′ ē ə loj′ ik) *physiological* (fiz′ ē ə loj′ i kəl) Each of these terms has a different suffix you have seen before.
-ology	**171** *Physi* is a root meaning "nature." The way that it is used here, it would be more accurate to say it means the "nature of (living things)," that is, the nature of body function. *Physiology* has the suffix ________, the same one found in *pelvology* (frame 56).
-ic -ical	**172** *Physiologic* contains the suffix ______, the same one found in *anatomic*, while *physiological* ends with the suffix ________, the same one found in *anatomical* (frame 74).
physi/ology physi/o/log/ic	**173** Subdivide *physiology*: ________/________, *physiologic*: ________/__/______/____,

physi/o/log/ical	and *physiological*: __________/__/__________/ ________.
Physiology	**174** ________________ is "the study of the nature" of living things or body functions. *Log* comes from the Greek for "study." It is actually a root, buried within the *-ology* suffix.
root	**175** In both *physi/o/log/ic* and *physi/o/log/ical*, *log* is a ________ (prefix/root/suffix). *Physi* is a root.
compound	**176** Both *physiologic* and *physiological* have two roots. Like *abdominopelvic* (frame 96) they are considered ______________ (simple/compound) words.
physiologic physiological	**177** Both ________________ and ________________ are adjectives "pertaining to the study of the nature of body function."
Physiological (Physiologic)	**178** ____________________("natural" body function) processes are closely regulated by *homeostasis* (hō′ mē ō stā′ sis, hō mē os′ tə sis).
-stasis	**179** *Homeo* is a root meaning "sameness." The only other word part in *homeostasis* is ____________. Therefore this word part acts as a suffix.
control of	**180** Go back and review Table 8, *Miscellaneous Suffixes*, in frame 55. You will see that *-stasis* means "________________."*

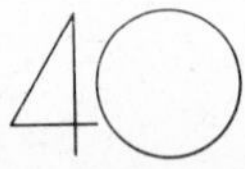

homeo/stasis	**181** Therefore ________/________ is a term indicating the "control of sameness" of body function.
homeostasis internal	**182** Without ________________ or regulation and maintenance of a high degree of "steadiness" of the body's ________________ ("inside") *environment*, life function as we know it would simply not be possible!

Now do the Self-Test for Unit 1 (page 261 in the Appendix).

UNIT 2
TERMS OF THE CELL

cells	**183** *Cell* comes from Latin and it means "compartment or chamber." The word was originally coined to describe the hollow ________ (compartments or chambers) visible as dark spaces in a piece of cork (Fig. 2.1).
	184 Observe and pronounce: *cellular* (sel′ yə lər) *extracellular* (eks trə sel′ yə lər) *intracellular* (in trə sel′ yə lər)
cellul	**185** The ending *-ul* means "small." Therefore, ________ is a root meaning "small chamber." You see that *-ul* here is not a suffix, but instead part of the root.
within (inside of) internal outside of (external; without)	**186** *Intra-* is a prefix meaning "________," the same as *en-* and *endo-* (frame 28). *Extra-* means the exact opposite of *intra-*, just as *external* is the exact opposite of ________. Consequently, *extra-* must mean "________ ________."*
cellul/ar intra/cellul/ar extra/cellul/ar	**187** Subdivide *cellular*: ________, *intracellular*: ________, and *extracellular*: ________

Table 2.1 ANATOMICAL TERMS OF THE CELL

cells	intracellular
cellular	lysosome
centrioles	microtubules
centromere	mitochondria
centrosome	mitochondrial
chromosome	mitochondrion
crista	nuclear
cristae	nucleolus
cytological	nucleus
cytology	organelle
cytoplasm	polyribosomes
cytoplasmic	ribosome
endoplasmic reticulum (ER)	rough ER
extracellular	smooth ER
Golgi	vacuole
granule	vesicle

cellul; -ar

________. The root in each case is ______ ______ and the suffix is ______.

Cellular

188

________________ is a term that "refers to a small chamber." In the bark of a cork tree these chambers are surrounded by rigid walls. Inside the human body each chamber is enclosed within a soft pliable *membrane* (mem' brān).

Intracellular

extracellular

189

________________________ fluid is located "within the cell," whereas ________________ ___________ fluid lies "outside the cell," bathing the cell membrane (Fig. 2.1).

190

Cyt is a root for "cell." Each of these terms includes *cyt*:

cytology (sī tol' ə jē)
cytological (sī tə loj' i kəl)

Cell or Cellul ("Small Chamber or Room")

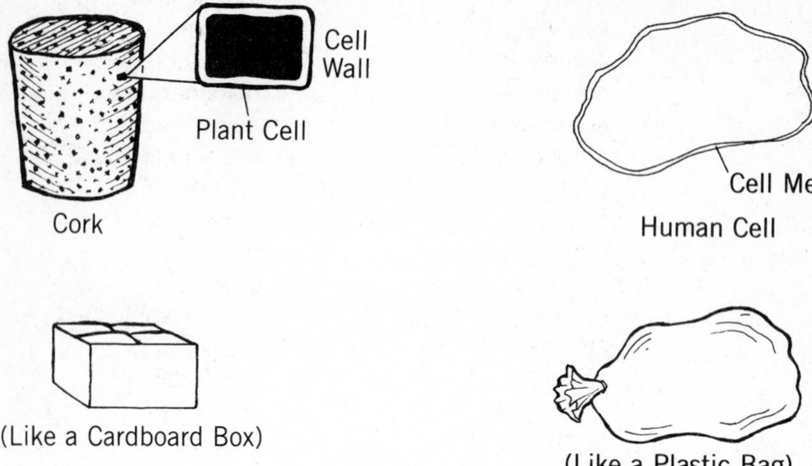

Figure 2.1. CELL VERSUS CORK

cytoplasm (sī′ tə plaz əm)
cytoplasmic (sī tə plaz′ mik)

191
Plasm is a root for "matter." You should now have sufficient information to divide these terms properly:

Answer	Frame
cyt/ology	*cytology*: _____/_________
cyt/o/log/ical	*cytological*: _____/__/_____/_______
cyt/o/plasm	*cytoplasm*: _____/__/_________
cyt/o/plasm/ic	*cytoplasmic*: _____/__/__________/____

192
Did you analyze all the terms correctly? If not, then review frame 173. After all, _________ _____ ("study of the cell") is divided the same way as *physiology*, and _________ _________ ("pertaining to study of the cell") is subdivided like *physiological*!

Answers: cytology; cytological

193
In both *cyt/o/log/ical* and *physi/o/log/ical*, the combining vowel __ connects the first root

Answer: o

log -ical	with ______, and the suffix in each case is ________. Isn't it ironic that this suffix means "pertaining to," just like *-ic* and *-al* separately?
Cytoplasm Cytoplasmic	**194** ________________ ("cell matter") is a fluid medium that occupies much of the cell interior. ____________________ ("referring to cell matter") activities include the production, packaging, and breakdown of vital chemicals.
Endo-	**195** ________, like *en-* and *intra-* (frame 186) means "inside of" or "within."
endo/plasm/ic (en dō plaz′ mik)	**196** Build a term that means "referring to (something) within matter." Omit the root for "cell" and use *endo-* as the prefix: ________/ __________/____. (Use the same format as in frame 194.)
cellul	**197** *Reticul* means "little network" in Latin. The *ul* in *reticul*, like the *ul* in __________ ("small chamber," frame 185) means "little" or "small." Again, *ul* is part of the root.
presence of	**198** The suffix *-um* means the same thing as the suffix appearing in *umbilicus* (frame 128). You learned earlier that *ili/um* means "presence of the flank." Therefore *-um* means "________ ____________."*
reticul/um (re tik′ yə ləm)	**199** Employ this suffix to construct ________ ____/____ ("presence of a little network").
Endoplasmic reticulum	**200** ____________________________________* "refers to the presence of a tiny network within

the matter" of the cell. Like a miniature river branching into many channels it carries materials from one area of the cell to another.

201

E R

Endoplasmic reticulum is certainly a mouthful to pronounce! Small wonder that it is often designated by __ __, using its initial letters in capitals!

202

tiny or miniature

The suffix *-elle* means about the same as *ul* in *reticul* and *cellul*. Thus *-elle* means "________________"* (huge or gigantic/tiny or miniature). (At this point you may want to review Table 8, frame 55.)

203

organ/elle (ôr gə nel')

It should now be easy for you to build ______ /________, a term for "tiny or miniature organ."

204

endoplasmic

reticulum

organelles

The ________________________________ ______* or *little network within* the cyto*plasm* is but one of many different intracellular ____ ______________ ("tiny organs") (Fig. 2.2).

205

Pronounce each of the following three terms:

nuclear (nyo͞o' klē ər)
nucleus (nyo͞o' klē əs)
nucleolus (nyo͞o klē' ə ləs)

206

nuclear

nucleus

By now you should be gaining some sophistication in word analysis. Of the three terms listed in frame 205, both ______________ and ______________ have the same root. (*Hint*: *ol* is handled like *ul* was in frame 197.)

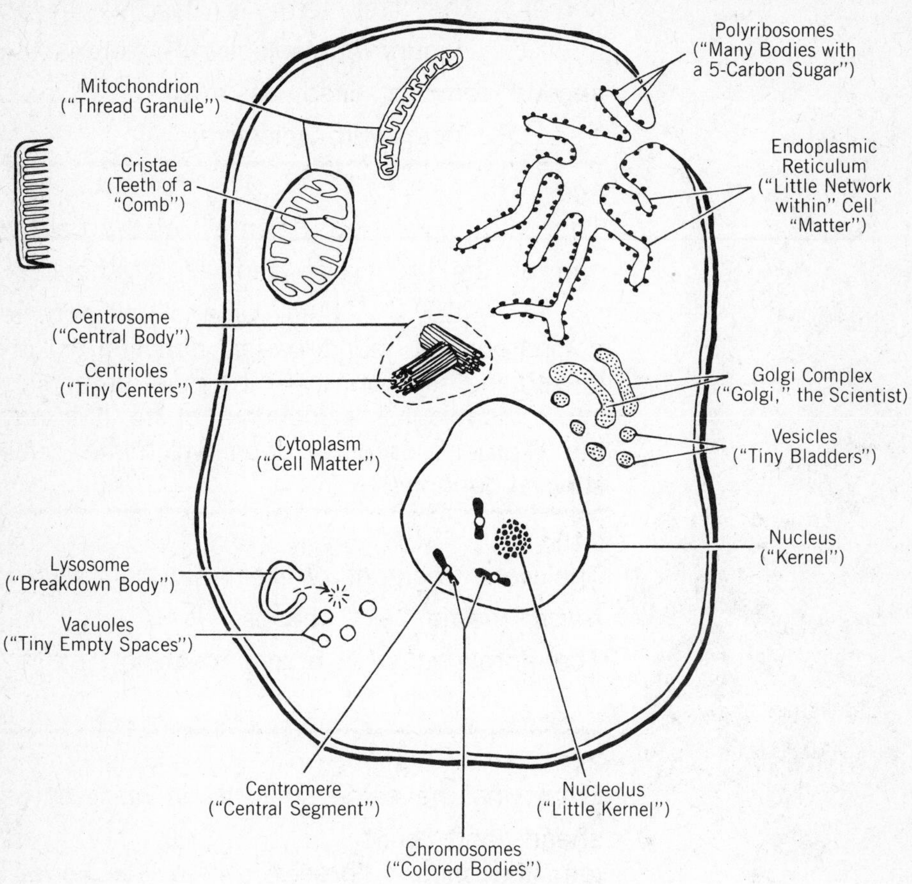

Figure 2.2. CELL ANATOMY

Answers	Frame
-ar -us nucle root	**207** How do we know this? First look for a familiar suffix in each term. The suffix in *nuclear* is ______, the same suffix found in *lumbar* (frame 123). The suffix in *nucleus* is ______, the same as the one in *umbilicus* (frame 120). The word part common to both *nuclear* and *nucleus* is then ________ ("kernel"), the ______ (main idea) in each case.
Nucle/us	**208** ________/____ means "presence of a ker-

nucle/ar

noun

adjective

nel," and ________/___ "pertains to a kernel." The first term is used as a/an ______ (noun/verb/adjective), whereas the second term is used as a/an ________ ______ (noun/verb/adjective).

---

nucleus

organelles

209
The __________ ("kernel" of the cell) is one of the most important of all the ___ __________ ("tiny organs"). It can be compared to a "band leader" directing or "orchestrating" the activity of the other organelles into a meaningful "symphony" of life. It is truly the "kernel," or core, upon which the cell's survival depends!

---

little (small)

little kernel

210
The word fragment *ol* like the *ul* in *cellul* or *reticul* (frame 197), means "__________." Therefore *nucleol* is a root meaning "______ ______________."*

---

nucleol/us

211
Employing the same suffix as in *nucleus*, go ahead and build __________/___, a term that means "presence of a little kernel" or just "a little kernel."

---

nuclear

nucleolus

212
Within the nucleus, deep to the ______ ____ ("pertaining to kernel") *membrane*, a ____________ ("little kernel") or two may be seen.

---

nucleolus

nucleus

213
The ______________ is "a little kernel" because it is small and often found within the larger __________ ("a kernel") (Fig. 2.2).

214
Observe and pronounce the following group of terms:

centrosome (sen′ trə sôm)
chromosome (krô′ mə sôm)
lysosome (lī′ sə sôm)
ribosome (rī′ bə sôm)
polyribosomes (pol ē rī′ bə sômz)

---

presence of a body

215
Note that all the terms in the previous frame contain *some* (sōm). *Some* contains the root, *som* ("body") and the suffix *-e* ("presence of"). Thus *som/e* means "____________ ____________."*

---

som

organelles

216
Som derives from the ancient Greek *soma*, "body." The Greeks were referring to the entire human body, and we still use ______ (root for "body") in this way. In addition, however, we utilize this root for many tiny "bodies" or ____________ ("miniature organs") within the cell.

217
There are thus a number of different types of *some* in the cell. We use various roots before *some* to identify these types. These roots are:

centr "central"	*lys* "breakdown"
chrom "colored"	*rib* "a 5-carbon sugar"

---

chrom/o/som/e

centr/o/som/e

lys/o/som/e

rib/o/som/e

218
Employing "o" as a combining vowel, build terms with the following meanings:

______/__/______/__ "presence of a colored body"

______/__/______/__ "presence of a central body"

______/__/______/__ "presence of a breakdown body"

______/__/______/__ "presence of a body" composed of a "5-carbon sugar"

Chromosomes nucleus	**219** ________________ ("colored bodies") are dark wormlike structures contained within the cell ________ ("kernel") (Fig. 2.2.) They contain most of the cell's hereditary material.
centrosome cytoplasm nucleus	**220** The ________________ ("central body") is a region of the ________________ ("cell matter") near the ________________ ("kernel") (Fig. 2.2). This organelle is involved in cell division.
lysosome organelle lyso cytoplasm	**221** The ________________ ("breakdown body") is an ________________ ("tiny organ") that contains digestive chemicals. When the ________ *-some* ruptures, these chemicals are released into the ________________ ("cell matter") and "break down" foodstuffs and other materials in the cell (Fig. 2.2).
ribosome intracellular	**222** A ________________ is a small dark "body" containing the "5-carbon sugar," *ribose* (rī' bōs). This tiny organelle is the site of most ________________ ("within cell") protein synthesis.
many	**223** *Poly-* is a prefix meaning "________." (Consult Table 5, frame 45).
poly/rib/o/som/es (pol ē rī' bə sōmz) endoplasmic reticulum	**224** Thus ________/________/__/________/____ are long chains of "many ribosomes" involved with protein synthesis. These chains are often located along the ________________ ________________* ("a little network within the matter" of the cell) (Fig. 2.2).

Rough
poly-
Smooth

225
Endoplasmic reticulum can have either a "rough" or a "smooth" surface. ________ (Rough/Smooth) *ER* is studded with ________ *-ribosomes*, giving it a rather coarse granular appearance. ________ (Rough/Smooth) *ER* lacks any such ribosome chain.

226
Examine and pronounce these terms:

microtubule (mī krō tyo͞o′ byo͞ol)
centriole (sen′ trē ōl)
centromere (sen′ trō mir)
vesicle (ves′ i kəl)
vacuole (vak′ yo͞o ōl)

Centriole
centromere
centr

227
________ and ________ are the two terms in frame 226 that contain ________, the root for "central."

---

centr/o/mere

228
-mere is a suffix denoting "segment." Thus a ________/__/________ is the "central segment" of a chromosome (Fig. 2.2). It splits apart during cell division.

---

ol

229
Recall from frame 210 that ____, contained within the root, *nucleol*, means "little" or "small." When placed after a root at the end of a term, this word fragment becomes the suffix, *-ole* ("tiny").

---

centr/i/ole

230
For example ________/__/______ is a term meaning "tiny center," where *i* is used as a connecting vowel.

Centrioles
centrosome

231
________ ("tiny centers") are located within the ________

chromosomes	("central body"), and they are thought to move apart and form a spindle or plate for the _____________ ("colored bodies") during cell division (Fig. 2.2).
ul	**232** Remember from frame 210 that ____ is the fragment in both *cellul* and *reticul* that means "little" or "small." When placed at the end of a term, it becomes the suffix *-ule* ("tiny"), as in *miniscule*.
micr/o/tub/ule	**233** *Micr* is a root meaning "tiny." Both the first root and the suffix in ________/__/______/ ______ (frame 226) mean "tiny." *Tub*, the second root, means "tube."
Microtubules cytoplasm centrioles	**234** _______________ are "tiny tubes" found within the _____________ ("cell matter"). They may assist in cell division, along with the _____________ ("tiny centers") of the centrosome.
-elle -ole; -ule	**235** You have now learned that _________, ________, and ________ are suffixes that mean "little, small, or tiny."
Vacuole	**236** _____________ is the other term in frame 226 that contains *-ole*. *Vac* is a root for "empty space," as in a *vacuum*.
Vac/u/ole	**237** ______/__/______ is a term meaning "tiny empty space." It contains the connecting vowel *u*.
vacuoles	**238** In actuality, _____________ within the cell are not "empty" at all. They commonly hold

lysosomes	food, air, or water, and are surrounded by a membrane. These structures are often digested by ________________ ("breakdown bodies") (Fig. 2.2).
vesic/le	**239** *Vesic* means "bladder." The term in frame 226 that contains this root is subdivided as __________/____.
-le	**240** If *vesicle* is a term meaning "little bladder," then ______ must be a suffix for "little."
-elle; -ole; -ule -le	**241** Now you have learned a total of four different suffixes, ________, ________, ________, and ______, that mean "tiny, little, or small."
Vesicles	**242** ________________ ("small bladders") within the cell are usually membrane-surrounded sacs that contain special products manufactured by the cell organelles.
Golgi	**243** The *Golgi* (gōl′ jē) *complex* is itself an organelle (Fig. 2.2). Its vesicles serve as storage depots for secretions before their release from the cell. __________ derives from Camillo Golgi, the Italian scientist who first described the tiny organ.
Golgi complex	**244** While the ___________________________* is important for cellular packaging and secretion, another organelle, described by the three terms below, is crucial for cellular energy production: *mitochondrion* (mī tō kon′ drē ən) *mitochondria* (mī tō kon′ drē ə) *mitochondrial* (mī tō kon′ drē əl)

mitochondrion -on	**245** Of these terms it is ________________ ______ that contains ______, a two-letter suffix indicating "presence of." (Consult Table 7, frame 51, if necessary.)
mitochondria	**246** Singular terms ending in *-on* generally take plural form with *-a*. Thus ______________ ________ means "more than one mitochondrion."
Mitochondrial -al	**247** ______________________________ in frame 244 contains ______, a suffix indicating "referring to" (Table 2, frame 30).
chondr	**248** *Mit* is a root for "thread," while __________ (frame 116) is a root for "cartilage," "gristle," or "granule." You should know that *gran/ule* is a "little grain," because it ends with *-ule*.
mit/o/chondr/i/on granule	**249** A ______/__/____________/__/____ ("presence of a thread granule") is an organelle that can assume a variety of different shapes. It can be long, thin, and rod-shaped, much like a narrow "thread." Or it can be more rounded in form, somewhat like a ______________ ("little grain") (Fig. 2.2).
Mit/o/chondr/i/al	**250** ______/____/______/____/______ ("pertaining to thread granule") functions include cell energy production.
crist/ae (kris' tē)	**251** *Crista* (kris' tə) means "comb" or "crest." Medical words ending in *-a* often have their plural using *-ae*. Therefore __________/____ are "combs."

crista

mitochondrial

252
Each ______________ ("comb") resides within a mitochondrion. It is actually a shelf-like projection of the inner ______________________ ("thread granule") membrane (Fig. 2.2).

cristae

253
As you can see from Figure 2.2, these ________________ all together do somewhat resemble the teeth of a "comb"! They are the sites of many important chemicals for energy production within the cell.

Table 2.2 PHYSIOLOGICAL TERMS OF THE CELL

adenosine diphosphate	genes	organic
adenosine triphosphate	genetic	osmosis
ADP	glucose	phagocytosis
anaphase	glycogen	phosphate
atom	hypertonic	pinocytosis
ATP	hypotonic	polysaccharide
ATPase	inorganic	prophase
biochemical	interphase	proteins
carbohydrate	ion	ribonucleic acid
chemical	isotonic	ribose
deoxyribonucleic acid	lipase	RNA
diffusion	lipid	saccharide
disaccharide	meiosis	semipermeable
DNA	metaphase	solute
electrolyte	mitosis	solution
element	molecule	solvent
	monosaccharide	telophase
	nucleic	tonic

organelles

254
The cell ______________________ ("tiny organs") function at the chemical level. Look at the definitions of these chemical terms:

element "a rudiment; beginning"
atom "indivisible; uncuttable"

element atoms	**255** An ____________ ("rudimentary" chemical) is the simplest, most basic form of a chemical. It consists of ________ ("indivisible" or "uncuttable" particles) of one kind only.
element atoms	**256** *Oxygen*, represented by the letter *O*, is a simple "rudimentary" ____________ consisting of many "indivisible" O ________ only.
tom a/tom	**257** Look closely at *atom*. It contains the root ____, the same one found in *anatomy* (frame 69). Subdivide *atom*: __/____.
a- a/tom	**258** The prefix in atom is simply ___, which means "not" or "without." You see that __/ ____ is a term meaning "not cuttable," since *tom*, the root, means "cut."
atom	**259** Over 2,000 years ago the Greek philosopher, *Democritus* (de mok′ ri təs), speculated that if matter were divided into smaller and smaller pieces, it would eventually reach a point where it was "uncuttable." This smallest bit of "uncuttable" matter he called the ______.
nuclear atom	**260** But with modern "atom-smashers" that can "cut" into atoms with high-energy beams, ____________ ("pertaining to the kernel," frame 208) physics has shown us that many smaller particles *do* exist within the ______ ("noncuttable" particle of matter)! So is this ancient term now inappropriate? What do *you* think?

261

atom
ion

Ions are simply atoms that have gained or lost smaller particles having electrical charges. The element *sodium* is represented as *Na*, the sodium ________ (atom/ion). But in the form Na^+, it is called an ______ (atom/ion) instead. This is because Na^+ has gained one net positive (+) charge.

262

ion
extracellular

Ion comes from the Greek for "going" or "carrying." For example Cl^-, the chloride ______, is "going" around in the ________________ ________ ("outside the cell," frame 189) fluid "carrying" a negative (−) electric charge.

263

-ule

Na^+ ion and Cl^- ion "go" together to form the NaCl or sodium chloride *molecule*. *Molecule* contains the root *molec* ("mass") and the suffix ________, the same suffix as in *microtubule* (frame 233).

264

Molec/ule

__________/______ must therefore mean "tiny mass."

265

molecule
atoms
ions

A ________________ ("little mass") is simply a combination of two or more __________ ("noncuttable" particles) or a combination of two or more ________ (charged atoms "going" places).

266

in-
-ic

Molecules can be either *organic* or *inorganic* in nature. *Organic* molecules contain the *carbon* (C) atom, whereas *inorganic* molecules do *not*. The ______ in *inorganic* must be a prefix meaning "not." And we find ______ at the end

	of both *organic* and *inorganic*, the same suffix as in *endopelvic* (frame 37).
Organ/ic carbon	**267** __________/____ literally means "pertaining to organs." This makes sense because all the *organs* in the body—heart, lungs, kidneys, and so forth—contain large quantities of ______ ______ (C) atoms!
6 0 organic inorganic	**268** The *glucose* (glo͞o′ kōs) molecule, $C_6H_{12}O_6$, contains __ (give the number) carbon atoms. The sodium chloride, NaCl, molecule, contains __(give the number) carbon atoms. Therefore students study about the glucose molecule during courses in ____________ (organic/inorganic) chemistry, and they learn about the sodium chloride molecule in ____________ (organic/inorganic) chemistry classes.
biochemistry in/organ/ic	**269** *Bio* means "life." Thus ______________ is the "chemistry" of "living" things. It includes both *organic* ("pertaining to carbon") and ____/ __________/____ ("not pertaining to carbon") chemical reactions.
a- in-	**270** In this unit you have learned that ____ and ______ are two prefixes meaning "not."
chemical (chemistry) chemical pertaining to	**271** *Chem* is a root probably meaning "________ ________." Surely you have already heard of ____________ ("pertaining to chemistry") reactions! The suffix in this case is *-ical*, which must mean "____________________"* (check back with Table 2, frame 30, for confirmation).

bio/chem/ical	**272** Build a term that means "referring to the chemistry of living things": ______/______/ ______.
biochemical molecule	**273** Most ______________ reactions of "living" things occur in a watery environment, either inside or outside the body cells. For example a sodium chloride (NaCl) or "common table salt" ____________(atom/element/ion/molecule) is broken apart and *dissolved* by the action of surrounding H_2O (water) molecules.
	274 Both *solv* and *solut* mean "dissolve," and they appear in such terms as these: *solvent* (sol' vənt) "one that dissolves" *solute* (sol' yo͞ot) "presence of the thing dissolved" *solution* "the act or process of dissolving"
solut/e solv/ent solut/ion	**275** In frame 274, ________/__ has the same suffix as *chromosome* (frame 218). According to frame 55 (Table 8), ______/_____ has a suffix meaning "one that," and ________/ _____ makes use of a suffix for "the act or process of."
solvent solute solution	**276** A __________ is a liquid "that dissolves" solid particles of ________ ("the thing that is present and is being dissolved"). And a __________ is the mixture formed by the "dissolving process." In other words, the *solution* is created by the dissolving action of the liquid *solvent* on the particles of *solute*.
	277 In the case of NaCl (common salt) and H_2O

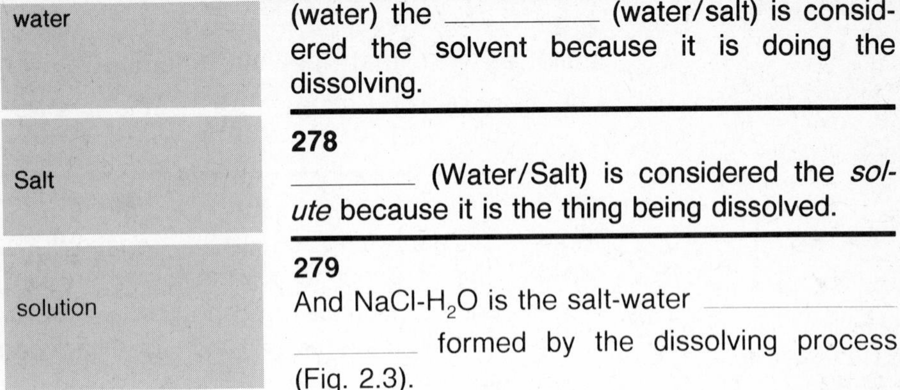

water	(water) the ________ (water/salt) is considered the solvent because it is doing the dissolving.
Salt	**278** ________ (Water/Salt) is considered the *solute* because it is the thing being dissolved.
solution	**279** And NaCl-H_2O is the salt-water ________ ________ formed by the dissolving process (Fig. 2.3).

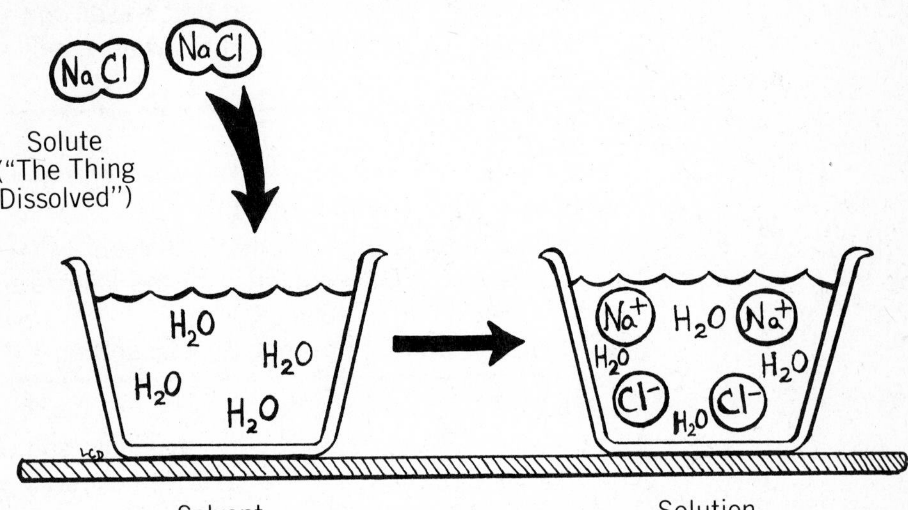

Figure 2.3. ***SOLUTES, SOLVENTS, AND SOLUTIONS***

ions	**280** Observe in Figure 2.3 that NaCl solute has been dissolved by interaction with water solvent into both Na^+ and Cl^- ________ (atoms/ions/molecules).
lys	**281** The sodium chloride molecule has been "broken down" into individual Na^+ and Cl^- ions. Recall that ______ is a root meaning "breakdown," as in *lysosome* (frame 217). And re-

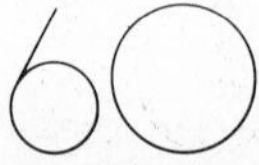

ion	member that ______ (frame 262) means "going" or "carrying."

282

These ions from "broken down" molecules "go to" areas of opposite electrical charge, the Na^+ ions attracted to ______________ (positively/negatively) charged areas, and the Cl^- ions attracted to ______________ (positively/negatively) charged regions. In so doing, such moving ions in water are capable of carrying an electric current.

negatively

positively

283

Electr/o represents the root for "__________ __________" and an appropriate combining vowel. *Lyt* (like *lys*) means "__________ ________," and it usually takes ____ as a "presence of" suffix, just the way *lysosome* does. An ________/__/______/__ is a substance that "breaks down" in water solvent and is capable of conducting "electricity."

electricity (electric)

breakdown; -e

electr/o/lyt/e (i lek′ trə līt)

284

NaCl is a common ______________ (electrolyte/nonelectrolyte). It is dissolved by water solvent and "broken down" into individual ______ and ______ ions. This type of charged solution is fully capable of conducting or "carrying" an electric current.

electrolyte

Na^+; Cl^-

285

In addition to their variable ability to conduct an electric current, solutions can be classified according to their "strength" or concentration of __________("the thing dissolved"). *Ton* is a root meaning "strength," and it generally combines with the suffix ______ to form an adjective. This is the same adjectival "pertaining to" suffix found within *endoplasmic* (frame 196).

solute

-ic

Ton/ic (ton' ik)	**286** ______/____ means "pertaining to (solute) strength." Observe and pronounce each of the terms below involving "strength": *isotonic* (ī sō ton' ik) *hypotonic* (hī pō ton' ik) *hypertonic* (hī pər ton' ik) Each term starts with a different prefix.
iso- hypo- hyper-	**287** According to Tables 4 and 5 (frames 42 and 45 in the *Word-Building* section), these prefixes are as follows: __________ "same; equal" __________ "below; deficient" (frame 114) __________ "above normal; excessive"
iso/ton/ic intracellular	**288** An ______/______/____ solution is an "equal strength" solution. By this it is meant that the concentration of solute in the solution is the "same" as the solute concentration of the ____________________ ("within the cell") fluid.
hypo/ton/ic	**289** A ________/______/____ solution is a "below strength" solution. In this case the concentration of solute in the solution is "below" or less than the solute concentration of the intracellular fluid.
hyper/ton/ic	**290** A __________/______/____ solution is an "above normal strength" solution. Here the concentration of solute in the solution is "above" the concentration of solute "normally" found in the intracellular fluid.
hypertonic	**291** The human red blood cell shrinks when placed into __________________ ("excessively con-

	centrated") solutions. It swells when placed into
hypotonic	________________ ("deficiently concentrated" or dilute) solutions. But it stays the
isotonic	"same" size when placed into ____________ ("equally concentrated") solutions. In other words, the cell will either expand or shrink in volume whenever the concentration of solute in the surrounding solution is not *equal* to the concentration of solute within the cell.

292

Cells change in size owing to the net loss or gain of particles passing through their membranes. Membranes that let particles pass through them are said to be *permeable* (pûr′ mē ə bəl). *Perme* is a root meaning "pass through." And *-able* is a suffix meaning "able." *Semi-* is a prefix for "partially." Thus a

semi/perme/able (semē pûr′ mē ə bəl)	________/__________/________ membrane is one in which particles are "partially able to pass through."

293

semipermeable	The cell membrane is ________________ ________, allowing certain particles to "pass through" it, while preventing or restricting the passage of others. The two most important means by which particles cross membranes are *osmosis* (oz mō′ sis) and *diffusion* (di fyo͞o′ zhən).

294

The roots in both these terms imply movement:

osm "thrusting"
diffus "spreading out" or "scattering"

condition of	The suffix, *-osis*, means "________________ ________"* (Table 8, frame 55). An *-on*
presence of	means "______________________,"* like the ending in *mitochondrion* (frame 245).

Diffus/i/on i	**295** ____________/__/____ is the "presence of a scattering or a spreading out" of particles from a region where their concentration is high to a region where their concentration is low. The letter __ is a connecting vowel in this term, just as it is in *mit/o/chondr/i/on.*
Osm/osis	**296** ______/________ is the "condition of thrusting" brought about by the diffusion of large numbers of *water* molecules from a region where their concentration is high to a region where their concentration is low. This process may contribute to the powerful upward "thrust" of growing plants!
Diffusion osmosis	**297** Both diffusion and osmosis involve the chance or random "scattering" of particles. This may occur across the cell membrane and possibly affect cell size. The real difference between these two processes lies in the nature of the particles that are "spreading out." ____________________ (Diffusion/Osmosis) could apply to almost any moving particle, whereas ______________ (diffusion/osmosis) involves the "scattering" of *water* molecules *only*!
-osis	**298** Many other terms besides *osmosis* contain the suffix ____________ ("condition of"). Observe and say these terms: *phagocytosis* (fag ō sī tō′ sis) *pinocytosis* (pī nō sī tō′ sis)
cell	**299** The roots in these terms are: *phag* "eat" *pin* "drink" *cyt* "________" (frame 190)

Phag/o/cyt/osis pin/o/cyt/osis	**300** _____/__/____/_____ is a "condition of cell eating," while ____/__/____/_____ is a "condition of cell drinking."
phagocytosis vacuoles pinocytosis	**301** White blood cells may consume bacteria by means of __________ (phagocytosis/pinocytosis) and form water ________ ("tiny empty spaces," frame 237) as a result of __________ (phagocytosis/pinocytosis).
organic	**302** Cells may consume sugars, fats, proteins, and other types of __________ ("pertaining to organs/carbon," frame 267) chemicals. Suffixes such as *-id* "belonging to a group" *-ide* "a chemical compound consisting of two different elements or parts" are often used in some of the names for these chemicals.
lip/id (lip′ id) sacchar/ide (sak′ ə rīd)	**303** *Lip* is a root for "fat" and *sacchar* means "sugar." The fats are classified in the ____/___ family because "fats belong to this group." The ________/____ family is the family of "sugar compounds consisting of two different parts."
lipids saccharides	**304** Both the ________ ("fat group" members) and the __________ ("sugars composed of two different parts") serve as important sources of body fuel.
-ide	**305** Why is the suffix _____ ("compound of two

glucose	different parts") used with *sacchar*? Let us look at one type of saccharide, ______ ______ ($C_6H_{12}O_6$, frame 268), as a specific example.
$C_6H_{12}O_6$	**306** Glucose, having the chemical formula ______________, could be considered as consisting of equal numbers of carbon (C) atoms and water (H_2O) molecules; that is, the chemical formula for it can be rewritten as $C_6(H_2O)_6$, six carbons and six waters!
saccharide H_2O	**307** Consequently glucose is a ______________ ______ because it is a "sugar composed of two different parts:" a *carbon* (C) part, and a *water* (______) part!
carb/o/hydr/ate (kär bō hī′ drāt, kär bō hī′ drət)	**308** The suffix *-ate* means "something that." *Carb/o* indicates "carbon" and *hydr* is the root for water. Thus ________/__/________/______ translates as "something that is carbon and water."
saccharides carbohydrate	**309** The ______________________ ("sugars with two different parts") are all members of the ______________________ (CH_2O or "carbon-water") family, since each of them consists of equal parts of *carbon* atoms and *water* molecules! Isn't this terminology getting beautifully precise?
	310 Terminology can indeed have the exactness of mathematics! For example, observe and pronounce the terms below involving prefixes of number or proportion: *monosaccharide* (mon ō sak′ ə rīd) *disaccharide* (dī sak′ ə rīd)

polysaccharide (pol ē sak′ ə rīd)

mono-
di-
poly-

According to Table 5, frame 45, in the *Word-Building* section, ________ is a prefix for "single," ________ for "double" or "two," and ________ for "many."

---

mono/sacchar/ide
di/sacchar/ide
poly/sacchar/ide

311
Glucose is a ________/________________/______, because it is a "single sugar" that cannot be broken down into any simpler type of sugar. *Sucrose* (common table sugar) is a _____/________________/______ because it can be broken down into "two" smaller types of "sugar" molecules. And *glycogen* (glī′ kə jən) is a ________/________________/______ because it is composed of "many" individual glucose "sugar" molecules strung together like beads on a string.

---

glyc/o/gen

312
Glyc/o means "sweetness" and *-gen* is a suffix for "produce." When ________/__/______ ("sweetness producer") is broken down into its many individual glucose subunits, a *sweet* taste of sugar is *produced*. (See Fig. 2.4.)

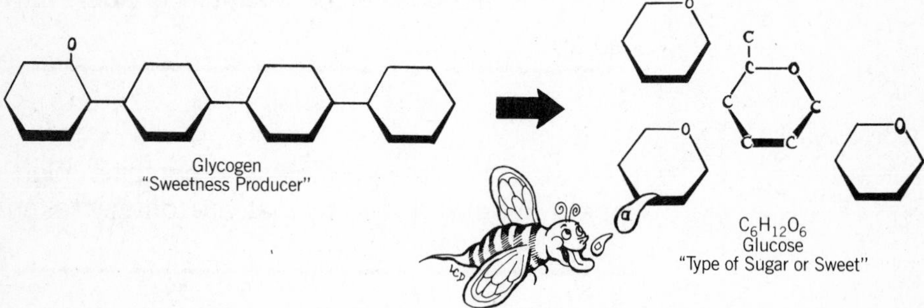

Figure 2.4. GLYCOGEN INTO GLUCOSE

313
Other chemical terms also involve prefixes of number:

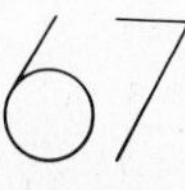

adenosine diphosphate (a den′ ō sēn dī fos′ fāt)
adenosine triphosphate (a den′ ō sēn trī fos′ fāt)

314
The *adenosine* molecule is a common ________________ (C-containing) molecule in the cell. Energy is required to attach one or more phosphorus atoms to this molecule.

organic

315
The suffix in *phosphate* is ________, the suffix also found within *carbohydrate*. *Phosphate* is analyzed as ____________/______, where ____________ is the root for "phosphorus."

-ate

phosph/ate

phosph

316
You would then expect *adenosine* ____/____________/______ to be "something that" contained "two phosphorus" atoms, while *adenosine* ______/____________/______ would be "something that" contained "three phosphorus" atoms. ________ is the prefix meaning "three."

di/phosph/ate

tri/phosph/ate

Tri-

317
If *a*denosine *di*phosphate is abbreviated as ADP, the *a*denosine *tri*phosphate is abbreviated as ______.

ATP

318
The ____________________________________ ____________* (ATP) molecule contains high-energy chemical bonds that are often broken to do cell work.

adenosine
triphosphate

319
The suffix *-ase* (ās) means "splitter." It simply follows whatever is being "split." Thus *ATP*-________ is the chemical that "splits" the ATP molecule, breaking one of its bonds and releasing the stored energy.

-ase

Answers	Frames
ATPase lip/ase (lip' ās)	**320** If __________ means "ATP splitter," then ______/______ must mean "fat splitter."
first	**321** Both ATPase and lipase are enzymes. Enzymes are proteins that speed up chemical reactions. *Protein* is a root meaning "first." Perhaps this is because proteins were probably one of the __________ (first/last) chemicals that became part of living things on earth.
Proteins ribosomes	**322** __________ ("first" chemicals) form the essential structure of all life. These crucial structural chemicals are produced by __________ ("bodies containing 5-carbon sugars," frame 218).
-gen	**323** Recall that ________ in *glycogen* (frame 312) is a suffix meaning "produce." This same word part can also serve as a root. For example, the *genes* direct the ribosomes to "produce" certain enzymes and structural proteins.
genet/ic	**324** *Genet,* like *gen*, is a root for "produce." Then ________/____ "refers to production," where the suffix is that in *hypertonic* (frame 290).
Genetic genes chromosomes nucleus	**325** __________ is an adjective that "pertains to the production" of enzymes and other types of proteins. The __________ ("producers") are tiny sections on the __________ ("colored bodies," frame 218) within the __________ ("kernel").
	326 These tiny chromosomal sections are com-

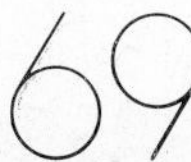

Answers	Frames
deoxyribo nucleic acid	posed of a chemical called *DNA*, or *deoxyribonucleic* (dē ok′ sē rī′ bō nyo͞o klē′ ik) *acid.* The *D* stands for ________________, the *N* for ________________, and the *A* represents ________.
Deoxyribonucleic acid nucle/ic	**327** ________________________________* (DNA) is one special type of ____________/____ ("referring to the kernel;" use *-ic*, not *-ar*) *acid.*
ribonucleic acid (rī′ bō nyo͞o klē′ ik)	**328** If *RNA* is the same as *DNA* except for the "D," then the long name for *RNA* is ________________________* rather than *deoxy*ribonucleic acid!
rib/o rib/o/nucle/ic	**329** Each term contains ______/__, one of the same roots and combining vowels found within *rib/o/som/e.* Analyze *ribonucleic*: ______/__/__________/__.
Rib/o	**330** ______/__ ("5-carbon sugar," frames 217, 218, 222) represents *ribose*, a specific chemical.
ribose nucleic	**331** Thus both DNA and RNA contain some form of ____________ (rib/o), and they are both ____________ ("pertaining to the kernel") *acids.*
RNA DNA; deoxy	**332** *Ribonucleic acid*, abbreviated by the three letters ______, differs from *deoxyribonucleic acid*, ______, in that it lacks __________ in its name.

Oxy de/oxy	**333** *De-* is a prefix that means "away from." ______ is the root for the element, *oxygen* (O). Then ____/______ means "an oxygen atom is taken away from." Take a guess! What do you think *deoxyribo-* means? (Examine Figure 2.5 carefully. How do the two molecules pictured differ?)

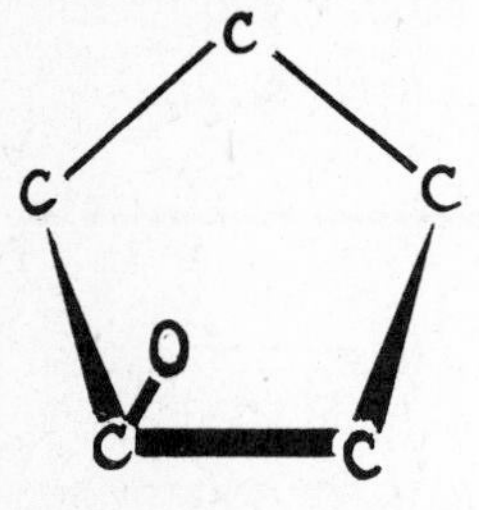

Ribose
("5-Carbon Sugar")
$C_5H_{10}O_5$

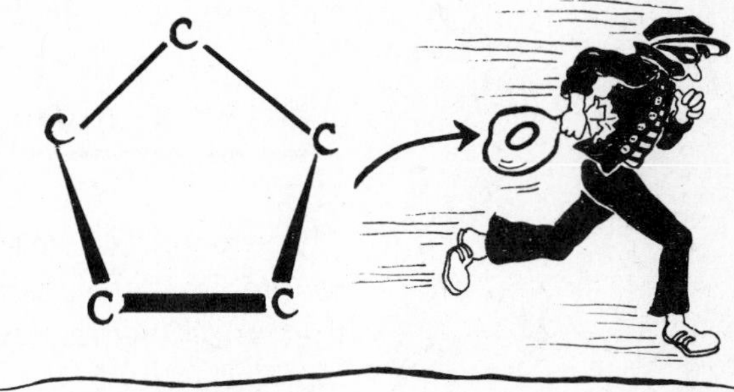

Deoxyribose
("5-Carbon Sugar with One O Taken Away")
$C_5H_{10}O_4$

Figure 2.5. RIBOSE VERSUS DEOXYRIBOSE

de/oxy/rib/o an oxygen atom (O) is taken away from the ribose	**334** Analyze *deoxyribo-*: ____/______/______/__. *Deoxyribo-* means "____."*
de/oxy/rib/o/nucle/ic	**335** A diagram of a ____/______/______/__/__________/____ acid molecule will show that it lacks an oxygen atom on each of its riboses. Hence the name *deoxyribo*nucleic acid!
nucleolus chromosomes	**336** RNA is found within the *ribo*somes and the ________________ ("little kernel," frame 211). DNA is primarily located within the ________________ ("colored bodies").

337

The *nucleolus* produces most of the cell's RNA. The *chromosomes*, containing the ________ ("producers") located along the length of their DNA molecules, provide the "blueprint" for much of the cell's activity.

genes

338

Both the *nucleolus* (mostly RNA) and the *chromosomes* (mostly DNA) are found within the ____________ ("kernel"). Hence both R*NA* and D*NA* are *n*ucleic *a*cids!

nucleus

339

Chromosomes within the nucleus somewhat resemble dark-colored "threads." But recall that another organelle, the *mit/o/chondr/i/on*, contains _____, the root for "thread." And you might also remember that *pinocytosis* (frames 298–300) contains the suffix ____ _____ ("condition of").

mit

-osis

340

Seeing that you are learning a word-building *system*, in which word parts from one term may be extracted and used with word parts from another term, it is just fine for you to build a new term, _____/_______ ("a condition of threads")!

mit/osis (mī tō′ sis)

341

Mei is a root meaning "lessening." Then _____/_______ is a term meaning "a condition of lessening."

mei/osis (mī ō′ sis)

342

Both *mitosis* and *meiosis* are forms of cell division, in which the chromosomes or "threads" divide and pull apart. From the meaning of their roots you can probably guess that ____________(mitosis/meiosis) is the "condition" of cell division in which the total num-

meiosis

mitosis	ber of chromosomes is "lessened" by one half, and that ______________ (mitosis/meiosis) results in no reduction in total chromosome number per cell.

343

Below are listed the prefixes used in naming the stages of both *mitosis* and *meiosis*. Some you may already know. Fill in their definitions with help from Table 4, frame 42:

up; toward; apart	*ana-*"______________________________"* (frame 71)
between	*inter-* "______________"
before; first	*pro-* "________________________"*
after	*meta-* "__________"
end	*telo-* "______"

344

Name each of the five different phases of cell division that are described below:

inter	__________/phase	phase "between" cell divisions
pro	__________/phase	"first" phase of cell division
meta	__________/phase	the second phase, occurring "after" the first
ana	__________/phase	chromosomes move "apart" to opposite ends of the cell
telo	__________/phase	the final stage that "ends" cell division

Now do the Self-Test for Unit 2 (page 263 in the Appendix).

UNIT 3
TERMS OF THE TISSUES AND SKIN

Answer	Frame
gross micr	**345** We have discussed a number of suffixes for "small, little, tiny." We have identified one root for "large." For example, ________ ("large") anatomy involves the study of structures visible to the naked eye. Most cells are quite small. Observe these roots for "large" and "small" below: *macr/o* "large" ___/*o* "small" (frame 233)
micr/o/scop/e (mī′ krə skōp) cyt	**346** *Scop* means "examine." A ________/__/________/__ is an instrument used to "examine small" things, like cells and tissues (collections of similar cells). Recall that ______ is the root for "cell."
hist/ology (his tol′ ə jē)	**347** *Hist* means "tissue" or "web." If *cyt/ology* is "the study of cells," then ________/____________ must be "the study of tissues or webs."
phag -e	**348** You may remember that ________ is the root within *phag/o/cyt/osis* (frames 299–300) that means "eat." This root, like *scop/e* and *centr/o/som/e* (frame 218) can take the suffix ____ ("presence of"). Try to build a term

Table 3.1 STRUCTURAL TERMS OF THE TISSUES AND SKIN

adipose	fibroblast	serous
areolar	fibrous	squamous
collagen	gland	strata
columnar	glandular	stratum
corium	histiocyte	stratum basale
cuboidal	histology	stratum corneum
cutaneous	hypodermis	stratum germinativum
cuticle	macrophage	stratum granulosum
cutis	microscope	stratum lucidum
dermis	microscopic	stratum spinosum
elastic	mucous	subcutaneous
epidermis	papilla	subdermis
epithelial	reticular	synovial
epithelium	sebaceous	
fascia	sebum	

macr/o/phag/e (mak′ rō̦ fāj)

meaning "presence of a large eater": ________/__/________/__.

349

Macrophages

________________________ are "large" cells that, like hungry spiders looking for something to "eat," migrate among the body tissues in constant search for foreign matter and cell debris.

350

web
cyt/e
histi/o/cyt/e (his′ tē ō sīt)

Histi/o, like *hist/o,* represents a root and combining vowel for "tissue" or "______." And ______/__ represents the root for "cell" and the same suffix as in *scope*. Build a term for "web cell": __________/__/______/__.

351

nucleol
areol/ar (a rē′ ə lər)

Areol is a root for "little area," just as ______________ (Unit 2, frame 210) is a root for "little kernel." And __________/____ is an adjective "referring to a little area," just as *nucle/ar* is an adjective "referring to a kernel."

Areolar	**352** __________ tissue is a particular type of connective tissue that contains many "little areas" between its fibers. It is also called "loose" connective tissue because it is a rather loose airy arrangement of cells, fibers, and the small spaces between them. (See Fig. 3.1.)
histiocyte macrophage areolar	**353** A __________ ("web cell") is usually defined as a __________ ("big eater") that is located within the "web" of loose __________ ("little areas") connective tissue (Fig. 3.1).
histiocyte phagocytosis	**354** A __________ (macrophage within loose areolar connective tissue) engages in the process of __________ ("cell eating"), thereby aiding in body defense.
fiber fibr/o/blast (fī′ brō blast)	**355** *Fibr/o* means "__________," while *blast* is a root for "sprout" or "forms," like a planted seed sprouting from the soil. So a ______/__/______ or "fiber-former" is a cell that produces or "sprouts" connective tissue fibers within areolar tissue like a spider spinning the silk strands of its web (Fig. 3.1).
Fibroblasts macrophages (histiocytes)	**356** __________ resemble spiders in that they form "webs" of fibers, while __________ resemble spiders in that they are "big eaters"!
	357 There are three different roots used to describe the different types of fibers commonly appearing within areolar tissue:

reticul

colla "glue"
elast "stretch"
________________ "a little network" (Unit 2, frame 197)

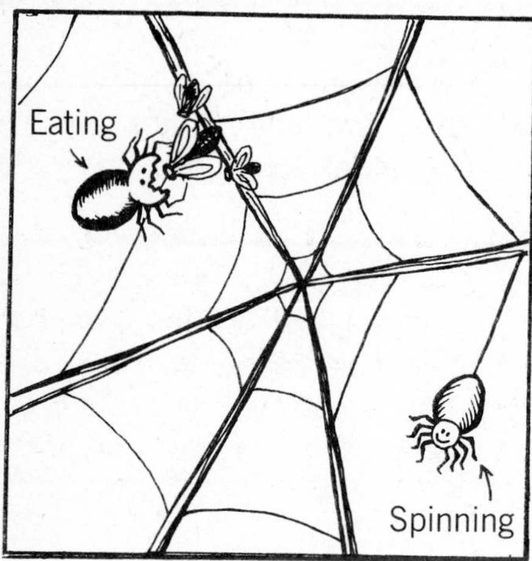

Web
Spider "Spinning" the Web Fibers, and Spider "Eating" Food

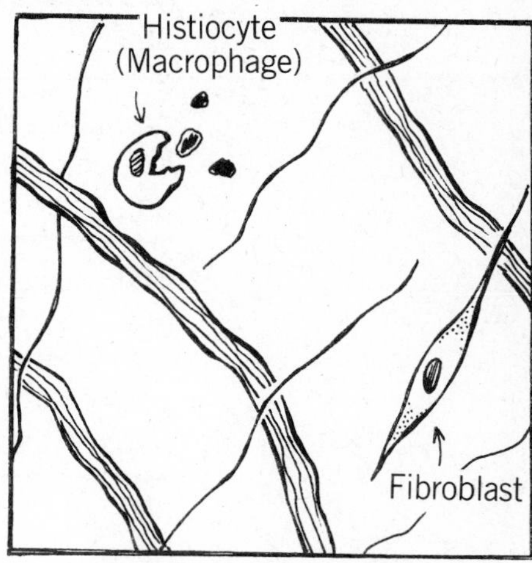

Areolar Tissue: ("Web of Little Areas"). Fibroblast "Spinning" Connective Tissue Fibers, and Histiocyte "Eating" Debris

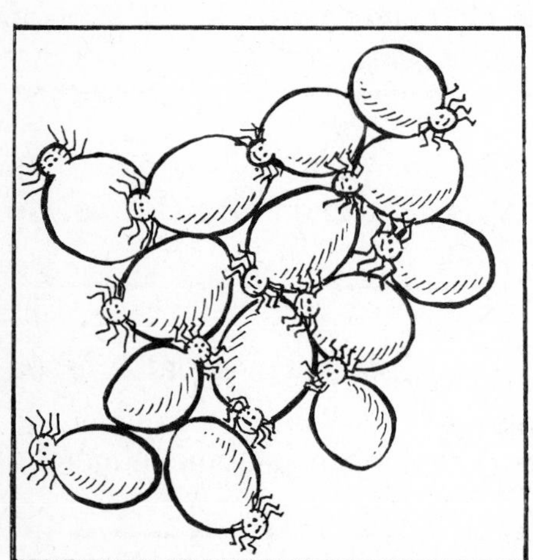
Fat Stuffed Spiders

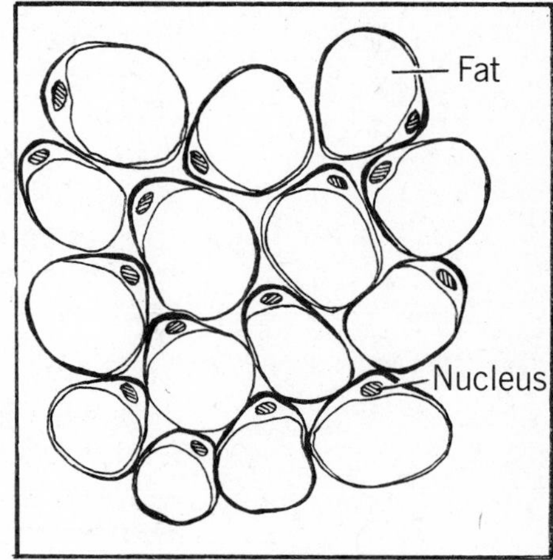

Adipose (Fat) Tissue (Adipose Cells Are Really Fibroblasts Stuffed with Fat)

Figure 3.1. TISSUE "WEBS"

gen colla/gen (kol′ ə jən)	**358** Remember that _____ means "produce" as in *gene* ("producer") and *glycogen* ("sweetness producer"). Here _________/_____ means "glue producer."
Collagen	**359** _______________ fibers are thick unbranched fibers that "produce" a firm "glue"-like stitching making steak tough and chewy to eat.
Elast/ic	**360** _________/____ fibers, just like the *elastic* in the waistband of a pair of pants, have the property of easy "stretchability," allowing connective tissue to be flexible and alter its form.
reticul/ar (re tik′ yə lər) -ar	**361** Finally _____________/____ or "pertaining to a little network" forms an adjectival suffix using _____, the same suffix found in *areolar*.
Reticular	**362** _______________ fibers are short "little" fibers forming a dense "network" of support for nerves, blood vessels, and cells.
lip	**363** *Adipos,* like _____ (Unit 2, frame 303), means "fat." This root often takes *-e* as the "presence of" suffix.
Adipos/e (ad′ i pōs) fibroblasts	**364** ___________/__ ("presence of fat") tissue basically consists of _______________ ("fiber-formers") that have become engorged with stored body fat.
adipose	**365** The cells in _____________ tissue somewhat resemble "fat" fully-fed spiders closely packed together! (Fig. 3.1.) And when body weight is lost some of the fat adipose-cell spi-

fibroblasts	ders become similar to "skinny" ________ ________ once more!
pertaining to	**366** *-Ous*, like *-ic*, *-al*, *-ar*, and *-ical*, is a suffix meaning "________________."*
Fibr/ous (fī' brəs)	**367** ________/______ ("pertaining to fibers") connective tissue forms a band or sheet covering various body structures. *Fasci* is a root for "band" or "sheet," and it takes *-a* as a "presence of" suffix.
Fasci/a (fash' yə) fibrous	**368** __________/__ ("presence of a band or sheet") forms a milky ____________ (mainly composed of "fibers") connective tissue film that covers much of the body beneath the skin.
fascia fascia	**369** Students performing dissection must often peel away the ___________, a fibrous connective tissue "sheet," before they can directly view the organs beneath. This is much like carpenters removing the wooden strip, "band," or ___________ covering the exposed edge of a roof overhang on a house. Who ever *said* that home construction and body construction have nothing in common!
fibrous	**370** Although fascia is primarily ___________ (fibrous/cellular) in nature, *epithelium* (ep i thē' lē əm) is just the opposite.
epi- -um	**371** *Theli* is a root for "nipple." The prefix in *epithelium* is ________, the same as for *epigastric* (frame 117). The suffix in *epithelium* is ______, just as it is in *reticulum* (frame 199).

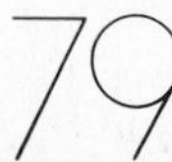

Epi/theli/um	**372** ______/____________/____ is a general type of tissue "present upon the nipples" and also upon many of the external and internal surfaces of the body.
epi/theli/al (ep i thē′ ē əl)	**373** Use the suffix in *distal* (frame 164) to build a term meaning "referring to (something) upon the nipples": ______/____________/____.
Epithelial	**374** ____________________ ("upon the nipple") tissue is cellular rather than fibrous in nature. The component cells may be shaped like cubes, columns, or scales. *Squam* means "scale," *cub* means "cube," and *column* means "column."
Squam/ous (skwā′ məs) diffusion osmosis	**375** __________/ ous ("referring to scales") epithelial cells are flat scale-like cells that form a thin barrier permitting ________________ ("spreading out," frame 295), ______________ ("condition of thrusting," frame 296), and filtration.
resembling	**376** *-Oid* is a suffix meaning "______________ ______" (Table 8, frame 55, in the *Word-Building* section). Strangely enough, the suffix *-al* is usually placed *after* this suffix when making a new term!
Cub/oid/al column/ar	**377** ______/______/____ ("cube-resembling") epithelial cells and ______________/ ar ("referring to column-shaped") epithelial cells are specialized for the function of secretion.
glandul	**378** *Gland* comes from the Latin for "acorn." If *cellul* is a root meaning "little chamber," then _______________ is a root for "little acorn."

gland
epithelial

379
A _________ ("acorn") is a collection of _________________ ("upon nipple") cells specialized for the job of secretion—releasing some useful product.

glandul/ar
(glan′ dyə lər)

380
The skin is one type of highly _______ _______/_____ ("pertaining to little acorns;" use the same suffix as in *columnar*) organ.

-ous
-um

381
Sebaceous (sə bā′ shəs) glands in the skin produce *sebum* (sē′ bəm) or "grease." *Sebaceous* ends with _______, the same suffix as in *fibrous*. And *sebum* terminates with _____, the suffix of *epithelium*.

seb/um
sebac/e/ous
seb
sebac

382
Sebum contains only one root + one suffix, while *sebaceous* contains one root + one combining (connecting) vowel + one suffix. Analyze *sebum*: ______/_____ and *sebaceous*: _________/___/______. The results of your analysis should convince you that both _____ and _________ are roots meaning "grease."

sebaceous
sebum

383
Overactive _________________ ("pertaining to grease") glands may contribute to the formation of pimples by clogging the pores with _________ ("a presence of grease").

papill/a (pa pil′ ə)

384
Papill is a root for "small pimple." This root takes the same "presence of" suffix as *fasci* (frame 367). Thus a ___________/__ is a "small pimple present" on the surface of the skin.

papilla

385
In modern usage, however, ___________

has come to represent any small nipplelike projection within the skin or elsewhere in the body.

386
Below are some different roots for "skin":

cori
cut
cutan
cutic
derm

Both *cut* and *derm* take ______ as their "presence of" suffix, the same way *pelv* (*Word-Building* section, frame 59) does. *Cori* forms a "presence of" noun with ______, just as *seb* (frame 383) does. And *cutan* forms a "pertaining to" suffix with combining vowel __ and ________, in a matter identical with *sebac* (frame 382).

-is

-um

e

-ous

387
________/______, ________/_____, and ______/_____ all mean "presence of the skin."

Cori/um; derm/is (kôr′ ē əm; dûr′ mis)

cut/is (kyo͞o′ tis)

388
You have learned that the prefix ________, means "upon." The ______/________/____ is a thin layer of epithelial cells "present upon the skin (*derm*)."

epi-

epi/derm/is (ep i dûr′ mis)

389
Recall that ______ in *vesicle* (frame 240) is a suffix meaning "little." Use *cutic* as a root to build a term meaning "little skin": __________ ____/_____.

-le

cutic/le (kyo͞o′ ti kəl)

390
The epidermis is also known as the ________ ______ ("little skin"), perhaps because of the extreme thinness of this topmost skin layer.

cuticle

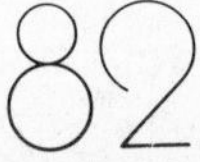

391

The *dermis* or ________/um or ________/is, the "true skin," is the deeper ________ ("referring to fibers") connective tissue layer of the skin. It is much thicker than the overlying ________________ ("presence upon the skin") or ______________ ("little skin").

Answers: cori; cut — fibrous — epidermis — cuticle

392

Recall that __________ (as in *hypogastric*, frame 114, Unit 1) is a prefix meaning "under" or "below." So is *sub-*.

Answer: hypo-

393

The ________/________/____ or the ______/________/____ is the region of fatty tissue "present" immediately "below the dermis."

Answers: hypo/derm/is (hī pō dûr′ mis) — sub/derm/is (sub dûr′ mis)

394

Of the five roots for "skin" given in frame 386, __________ is the one that combines with e/ous to make a "pertaining to" adjective. We can employ this root and *sub* to build a term meaning "pertaining to (something) beneath the skin": ______/__________/__/______.

Answers: cutan — sub/cutan/e/ous (sub kyo͞o tā′ nē əs)

395

If the "skin" is considered to be the *dermis* + the *epidermis* then the ________________ or ________________ (two terms for "below dermis") can be considered the fatty ________________________ ("beneath the skin") region immediately underlying the entire organ.

Answers: hypodermis — subdermis — subcutaneous

396

Above the dermis, there are a number of cell layers within the epidermis. *Strat* means "layer" or "bed cover." __________/____ means "presence of a layer or bed cover" just as *sebum* means "presence of grease."

Answer: Strat/um (strā′ təm)

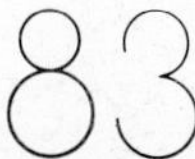

strat/a (strā′ tə)

397
Terms whose singular ends with *-um* form plural endings with *-a*. Then the plural of *stratum* must be __________/__.

strata

398
Like the "layers" of rock upon the earth or successive piles of blankets, sheets, and other "bed clothes" upon a mattress, successive __________ of epithelial cells form the epidermis of the skin.

stratum

little grain

399
Each __________ ("layer") has its own characteristic features and cell types. Note the meanings of the following roots involved with epithelial strata:

bas "base" or "bottom"
corne "horny"
granulos "__________________"*
(frame 249)
lucid "clear"
germinativ "sprout"
spinos "spine" or "thorn"

corne/um (kôr′ nē əm)
lucid/um (lyo͞o′ si dəm, lo͞o′ si dəm)
granulos/um (gran yə lō′ səm)
spinos/um (spī nō′ səm)

400
Each of the roots except *bas* in frame 399 takes *-um* as its "presence of" suffix. *Bas* takes *a/le*. Using this information, write the name of each layer of epithelium within the epidermis opposite its description below:

strat/um __________/____ the outer *horny layer*

strat/um __________/____ the *clear layer*

strat/um ______________/____ the *layer* containing cells with *small grains*

strat/um __________/__________ the *layer* whose cells are covered with *spines*

bas/a/le (ba sā′ lē, ba sal′ ee)

germinativ/um (jûr mi nə tī′ vəm)

strat/um ______/__/____ the deepest layer, forming a *little base*

strat/um ______________/____________ actually several *layers* from which most of the cells of the epidermis arise by *sprouting* (*mitosis*)

---

corneum

401
When we say that the stratum ________ ______ is "horny," we mean that it is imbued with a tough waterproof substance much like that found in the *horns* of animals!

---

spinosum

basale

germinativum

mitosis

402
Both the stratum ______________ ("spiny layer") and the stratum ____________ ("bottom layer, forming the base") are often included together under the name stratum ________ ____________ ("sprouting layer"). This is chiefly because these two deepest strata give rise to the upper strata by frequent ________ ______ (cell division involving no reduction in number of chromosomes).

---

external

cutan/e/ous

403
Remember that the epidermis is simply the ______________ ("outer") portion of the _________/__/_____ ("pertaining to skin," frame 394) membrane, the largest organ in the body!

404
Some other epithelial membranes also have highly specialized functions and locations. Look at these two roots for epithelial membranes:

muc "slime"
ser "whey" (the clear watery by-product of cheesemaking)

-ous

Both of these roots form a "referring to" suffix with ______, as in *fibrous*.

Ser/ous (sir′ əs)

muc/ous (myo͞o′ kəs)

405

Employ the information of frame 404 to complete the following statement: "__________/______ ('referring to whey') membranes line the closed body cavities and secrete a clear watery fluid, while ______/______ ('slime') membranes line the open body cavities and secrete a *slimy* sticky fluid."

---

mucous

406

When you blow your nose, __________ (mucous/serous) fluid appears in your kleenex, since the nose is part of a body cavity open and exposed to the air.

---

syn/ovi/al

(si nō′ vē əl)

407

Another type of membrane contains *ovi*, a root for "egg." *Syn-* is a prefix meaning "together." Build a new name for a membrane by using these word parts plus *-al*: ______/______/____.

---

synovial

408

This may seem odd, but __________ ("eggs together") membranes secrete a transparent fluid that resembles raw *egg* white! It is as if many *eggs* were cracked and their raw whites poured *together* into the cavities of moveable joints, serving to lubricate the bone surfaces and decrease the friction!

---

micr/o/scop/ic

(mī krə skop′ ik)

409

In closing, we can say that in addition to the ______/__/______/____ ("pertaining to examining small things," frame 346; use *-ic*) membrane of the individual cell, there are four different types of membranes involving sheets of cells:

cutaneous	____________	("skin") membranes
mucous	____________	("slime") membranes
serous	____________	("whey") membranes
synovial	____________	("eggs together") membranes

Now do the Self-Test for Unit 3 (page 267 in the Appendix.)

UNIT 4
TERMS OF THE SKELETON (CARTILAGE, BONE, AND JOINTS)

little	**410** Consider these roots: *ax* "axle; axis" *skelet* "dried body" *appendicul* "__________ (big/little) attachment"
Appendicul reticul	**411** ______________ ("little attachment"), like ____________ ("little network," frame 357), has its "pertaining to" format with *-ar*.
ax/is	**412** Picture a globe of the earth rotating on its ____/____ ("presence of an axle"). The globe itself is a hard "dried body" of wood or plastic.
skelet/on skelet/al	**413** The __________/____ is the hard "dried body present" after degeneration and disappearance of other organs and soft parts. It consists mainly of bones. Human __________/____ ("pertaining to dried body;" use *-al*) remains can be compared to the hard mass of a classroom globe.

Table 4.1 GENERAL SKELETAL TERMS

appendicular	diarthrosis	matrix
arthrosis	endochondral	medullary
articular	endosteum	osseous
axial	epiphysis	ossification
axis	Haversian	osteoblast
bursa	hyaline	osteoclast
canaliculi	intracartilaginous	osteocyte
canaliculus	intramembranous	periosteum
cartilaginous	lacuna	skeletal
chondral	lacunae	skeleton
chondrocyte	lamella	synarthrosis
diaphysis	lamellae	

414

axis

ax/i/al (ak′ sē əl)

The skeleton, like the globe of the earth, has a central ________, a line about which the structure could turn or revolve, like the axle of a wagon wheel. Use the appropriate root and *-i/al* to complete this statement: "The ____/ __/____ skeleton chiefly consists of the bones of the head, backbone, and rib cage. It forms the main axis or pivoting point in the center of the body."

415

axial

appendicul/ar (ap ən dik′ yə lər)

The skeleton, like pins stuck into a globe, has "little attachments" to its main ________ ("referring to axle") mass. This ________ ________/____ portion of the skeleton includes the bones of the shoulders and arms, as well as those of the hips and legs. In short, it includes all the bones that are *appended* or "attached" to the main body axis.

416

appendicular

Of course, both the axial and the ________ ________ skeletons are composed of bony tissue. Each of the following means "bone":

osse
ossi
oste/o

417

Now look at some other roots often used with *oste/o*:

Answer	
blast	_____ "sprouts" or "forms" (as in "fiber-former," frame 355)
	clast "break"
cyt	_____ "cell"

The root for "cell" usually takes *-e* as its "presence of" suffix.

418

Using the information provided in frames 416 and 417, test your skills as a word-builder: _______/__/_________ a "bone-producing" cell, _______/__/______/__ a mature "bone cell," _______/__/_________ a "bone-destroying" cell.

Answers: oste/o/blast (os′ tē ō blast); oste/o/cyt/e (os′ tē ō sīt); oste/o/clast (os′ tē ō klast)

419

While _________ is a root for "break," *fic* is a root for "make." This root generally follows *ossi*. Then _______/______ is an incomplete word fragment meaning "make bone."

Answers: clast; ossi/fic

420

Fic usually uses *a* as its connecting vowel with a suffix. Just such a suffix is *-tion*, which means "_______________________________." * Note that this is exactly the same meaning for _______, the suffix found in *solution* (frame 275).

Answers: the act or process of; -ion

421

Employ the word fragment of frame 419 and the facts in frame 420 to build a term that

ossi/fic/a/tion (os i fi kā′ shən)	means "the act or process of making bone": ________/______/__/________.
-ous osse/ous (os′ ē əs)	**422** *Osse* utilizes ________, the suffix in *fibrous*, to result in ________/______: "pertaining to bone."
Ossification osteoblasts osteocytes osteoclasts osseous	**423** ____________________ ("the process of bone formation") involves the gradual transformation of __________________ ("bone-forming" cells) into ________________ (mature "bone cells"). And ____________________ are large cells that help to remove or "break" preexisting ____________ ("bony") tissue, thereby assisting in remodeling the shape of bones.
chondr	**424** There are two basic types of ossification, one occurring "within cartilage" and one occurring "within a membrane." Below are two roots for "cartilage": *cartilagin* "cartilage" ____________ "cartilage, gristle, or granule" (frame 248) The root for "membrane" is simply *membran*.
-ous -al	**425** Both *cartilagin* and *membran* use ________ for "referring to," the suffix found within *osseous*. *Chondr*, on the other hand, combines with the suffix ______, as does *ovi* in *synovial* (frame 407).
cartilagin/ous chondr/al	**426** Thus both ______________/______________ and _____________/____ are terms that "refer

Answer	Frame
membran/ous	to cartilage," while ______/______ "refers to a membrane."
intra- endo-	**427** *Cartilagin* and *membran* combine with ______, the prefix in *intracellular* (frame 186), but *chondr* joins with ______, the prefix in *endoplasmic* (frame 196).
endo/chondr/al (en dō kon′ drəl) intra/cartilagin/ous (in′ trə kär ti laj′ i nəs)	**428** Putting all the information in the last four frames together, we have either ______/______/____ or ______/______/______ meaning "pertaining to (something) within cartilage."
intra/membran/ous (in′ trə mem′ brə nəs)	**429** Likewise, ______/______/______ "refers to (something) within a membrane."
endochondral intracartilaginous intramembranous	**430** The long bones of the arm and leg form by ______ or ______ ossification occurring *within* pre-existing *cartilage.* But the flat bones of the skull form by ______ ossification *within* large fibrous *membranes.*
osteoblasts osteocytes	**431** Whatever the exact manner of ossification, the ______ ("bone-formers") always assist in the production of a rock-hard *matrix* (mā′ triks) between cells. *Matrix* oddly means "a breeding animal" in Latin! Perhaps this strange analogy is made because in a sense the ______ (mature "bone cells") are "bred" from *osteoblasts* that have enclosed themselves within a white rock-

matrix

hard background substance called the ______________.

---

matrix

lacun/a (la kyōō′ nə)

432
But each osteocyte within the ______________ ("breeder") is surrounded by a small pool or "lake" of fluid. *Lacun* means "small lake," and ______________/__ is interpreted as "presence of a small lake," where *-a* is the "presence of" suffix.

---

lacunae (la kyōō′ nē)

433
The plural of *lacuna* is ______________, just as the plural of *crista* (Unit 2, frame 251) is *cristae*.

---

lacunae

434
Clopton Havers, an early English anatomist (1650–1702), must have had a vivid imagination when he looked through the microscope and described the small fluid-filled pits surrounding osteocytes as ______________ (Fig. 4.1)!

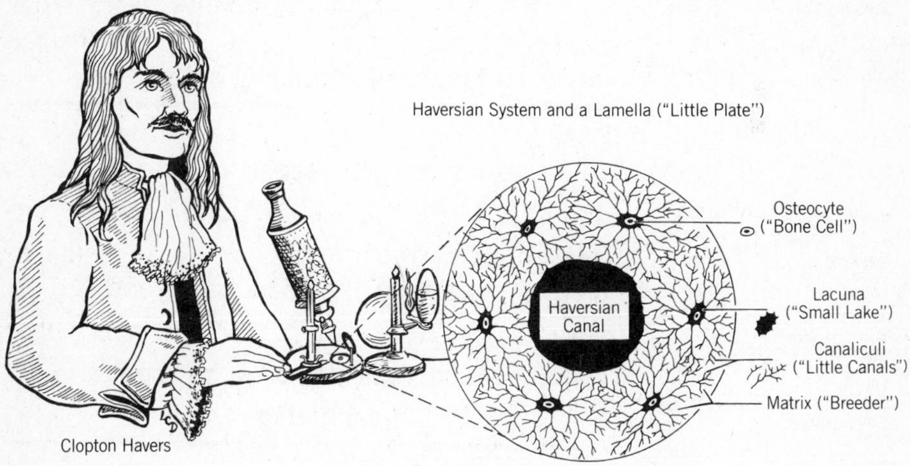

Figure 4.1. THE HAVERSIAN SYSTEM

---

lacunae

435
These ______________ ("small lakes") occur in rings around a large central hollow space

Haversian Havers	called the *Haversian* (ha vûr′ zhən) *canal*. This __________ canal is named for the English anatomist, Clopton __________.
little canals	**436** Clopton was a very clever fellow. See if you can follow his analogy! Look at Figure 4.1. What Havers described as *canaliculi* (kan ə lik′ yə lī) you would probably interpret as "______ __________"* in common English!
canalicul/us (kan ə lik′ yə ləs) lacuna osteocyte	**437** Scientific terms whose singular ends with *-us* generally have plurals ending in *-i*. Use this information to respond in the following sequence: "A __________/____ is a microscopic *canal* or channel connecting the __________ ('small lake') of one ______ __________ ('bone cell') with that of another lying adjacent to it."
Canaliculi lacunae	**438** __________ extend like small creeks between the __________ ("small lakes") surrounding individual osteocytes.
osteocytes matrix canaliculi Haversian	**439** Like islands of life afloat in watery lakes, __________ ("bone cells") are landlocked by rock-hard __________ (background substance between cells) and fed by tiny __________ ("channels") that eventually connect to a large central ____ __________ canal (Fig. 4.1).
lacunae	**440** The osteocytes in their __________ occur in concentric rings around each central Haversian canal. These circular rings of interconnected cells form "little plates" of matrix

little plates	between them. These "______________________"* are called *lamellae* (la mel′ ē).
Lamell/a (la mel′ ə)	**441** ___________/__ is the singular of *lamell/ae* just as *lacun/a* is the singular of *lacun/ae*.
lamella osseous	**442** Each ______________ is essentially a "little" curved "plate" of white ____________ ("bony") matrix that forms a ring around a central Haversian canal (Fig. 4.1).
lacunae canaliculi lamellae Havers/i/an	**443** Individual osteocytes lying within __________ (watery pits), interconnected via _________________________________ ("tiny channels"), and forming concentric ________________ ("little" circular "plates" of bony matrix) around a large central canal, together constitute a ____________/__/___ ("referring to *Havers*") *system* (Fig. 4.1).
pertaining to -an	**444** Haversian systems occur within the hard compact areas of bone, external to the inner marrow or *medullary* (med′ yə ler ē) cavity (Fig. 4.2). The suffix *-ary* means "__________________________,"* just like *-ar*, *-al*, *-ac*, *-ic*, *-ical*, *-ous*, and ______, the suffix in *Havers/i/an*.
Medull medial medull/ary	**445** _____________ (the root in *medullary*) sounds somewhat like *middle* or _____________ ("referring to the middle," frame 154). Thus _____________/______ is an adjective referring to the *medulla* or "middle" of a bone wherein the soft "marrow" lies.
medullary	**446** The ____________________ ("pertaining to mid-

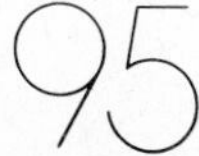

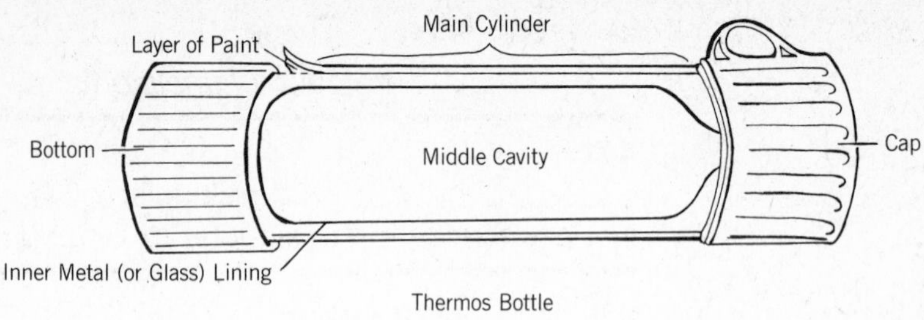

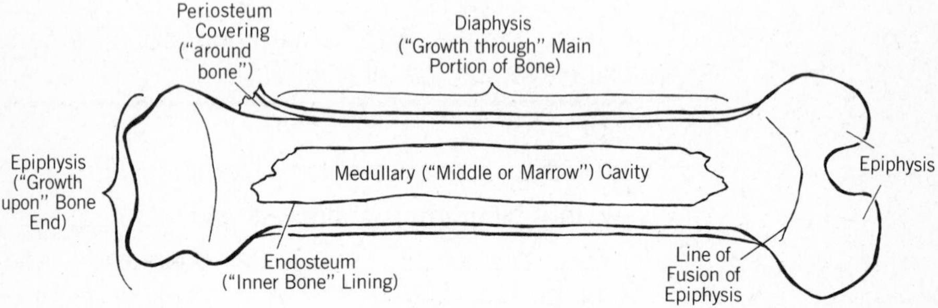

Figure 4.2. LONGITUDINAL SECTION OF A LONG BONE

endo-

-um

Oste

dle or marrow") cavity is lined by an *inner* membrane. Recall that __________ (frame 28, *Word-Building* section) like *en-* and *intra-* is a prefix meaning "inside of" or "within." And remember that ______, the suffix in both *corium* (frame 386) and *sebum* (frame 383) means "presence of (something)." _______, the root in *osteoblast* for "bone," can be combined with these two word parts.

End/oste/um
(en dos′ tē əm)

447

______/________/____ therefore means "presence of a (lining) within bone," where the terminal *o* on *endo-* has been dropped for easier pronunciation.

---

endosteum

448

The ________________ provides an inner membranous lining for the marrow present in the middle of a long bone, much as the metal lining of a thermos bottle envelopes the contents within.

449
According to Table 4 (frame 42, *Word-Building* section) *peri-* is a prefix meaning "__________." Using the same root and suffix as *endosteum*, build a term that means "presence of a (covering) around bone": ________/________/____.

around
peri/oste/um
(per ē os′ tē əm)

450
The ____________________ is a membrane "around" an entire long "bone," except for the bone ends. It can be peeled off the bone surface like paint from the sides of a metal thermos bottle (Fig. 4.2).

periosteum

451
Observe and pronounce the following two terms:

diaphysis (dī af′ i sis)
epiphysis (e pif′ i sis)

Each term is alike in that each contains ______, the "presence of" suffix within *pelvis* (frame 59). ________, the prefix in *epithelium* (frame 117) and in *epigastric* (frame 117), means "upon." According to Table 4 (frame 42, *Word-Building* section) ________ is a prefix for "through." And *phys* is a root meaning "growth."

-is
Epi-
dia-

452
Using the preceding information, fill in the blanks of this sequence: "The ______/__________/____ is a 'growth that is present through' the main length of the bone; that is, it is the main bone shaft. Conversely, an ______/________/____ is a 'growth present upon' each end of a long bone" (Fig. 4.2).

dia/phys/is
epi/phys/is

453
Like the *dia*meter of a circle or the main cylinder forming the long middle section of a

diaphysis	thermos bottle, the ______________ runs "through" the central portion of a long bone.
epiphysis	**454** And the ______________ upon each end of a long bone is somewhat like the bottom or cap upon the end of a long thermos bottle (Fig. 4.2).
epiphysis	**455** Each ______________ ("presence of a growth upon" bone) usually forms a joint with the end of some other bone. Both these roots involve joints: *articul* "little joint" *arthr* "joint"
articul/ar (är tik′ yə lər)	**456** Use the suffix *-ar* to complete the following statement: "The epiphysis of a long bone usually forms an ______________/____ ('pertaining to little joint') contact with another bone."
articular	**457** The ______________ or "little joint" surface of each bone epiphysis is covered with a layer of *hyaline* (hī′ ə lin) cartilage.
hyal/ine	**458** *Hyal* comes from the Greek for "glass." Thus ________/______ is a term that "refers to glass," where *-ine* is the "referring to" suffix.
Hyaline matrix lacunae	**459** ______________ ("glassy") cartilage has a smooth pearly ______________ ("breeding animal," frame 431) between the individual cartilage cells in their ______________ ("small lakes," frame 435).
chondr chondr/o/cyt/e	**460** Recall that ______________ (frame 116) is the root for "cartilage." Each ______________/__/

(kon′ drō sīt) lacuna	______/__ (mature "cartilage cell"), like each *oste/o/cyt/e* (mature "bone cell," frame 418) lies within a __________ ("small lake").
articular epiphysis hyaline	**461** The ______________ ("little joint") surface of each ______________ ("presence of a growth upon") of a long bone is capped by smooth glassy ___________ cartilage.
arthr hyaline	**462** Recall from frame 455 that ________ is a root for "joint." The ends of two different bones forming a freely movable joint are normally covered by a layer of ___________ ("glassy") cartilage, making the contacting bone surfaces as smooth as polished glass!
arthr/osis mei/osis -osis	**463** An ________/_______ is a "joint condition" just as _____/______ (Unit 2, frame 341) is a "condition of lessening." In each case the suffix is ________, "condition of."
di/arthr/osis syn/arthr/osis di- syn-	**464** Observe and pronounce the following two terms: *diarthrosis* (dī är thrō′ sis) *synarthrosis* (sin är thrō′ sis) The first is subdivided as ___/________/ ______, and the second as _____/___ _____/______, where _____ (as in *disaccharide*, frame 310) means "double" or "two," and ______ (as in *synovial*, frame 407) means "together."
suture synarthrosis	**465** A __________ ("seam," frame 147) between adjacent skull bones is one example of a ___________________ ("together joint

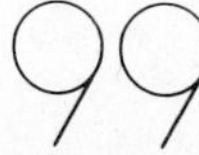

fibrous

condition"). This type of joint is considered immovable, because the *joining* bones are held tightly *together* by strong ______________ ("pertaining to fibers," frame 367) connective tissue.

---

diarthrosis

466

The knee joint is an example of a ________ ______________ ("double joint condition"), because the joint is so freely movable that it behaves somewhat like "double" joints or "two" joints rather than one! Such joints often have a *bursa* (bûr' sə) near them.

---

burs/a

467

Burs means "leather sac" or "purse." A ________/__ is a tough "leathery sac present" like a protective "purse" between moving structures where friction is likely to develop.

Table 4.2 TERMS OF SELECTED BONES AND MARKINGS

acromion	ethmoid	pterygoid
atlas	foramen	scapula
axis	fossa	sella turcica
capitulum	glenoid	sphenoid
cervical	humerus	sternum
condyle	hyoid	styloid
coracoid	mastoid	temporal
coronoid	nutrient	trochlea
cribriform	odontoid	vertebra
crista galli	pisiform	xiphoid
dens	process	xyphoid
epicondyle		

---

cervic/al (sûr' vi kəl)

vertebr

vertebr/a (vûr' tə brə)

468

Cervic means "neck" and ____________/ ____ "refers to the neck," just as *dors/al* "refers to the back." You might remember that ______________ (Unit 1, frame 102) is the root for "jointed backbone." Then __________ ______________/__ means "presence of a jointed backbone," just as *burs/a* means "presence of a leather sac or purse."

469

cervical vertebra

The first ______________________________ * ("jointed backbone" in the "neck") is called the *atlas*. In ancient Greek mythology Atlas was the god who supported the world on his shoulders.

470

cervical
cephalic
vertebral
atlas

Early anatomists cleverly used this myth to name the first ______________ ("neck") vertebra. This most ______________ ("pertaining to the head," Unit 1, frame 136) bone of the ______________ ("referring to jointed backbone," frame 106) column is called the __________. Obviously, this is because it supports the "world" of the skull on its "shoulders," in much the same way that the Greek god supported planet Earth in the heavens (Fig. 4.3).

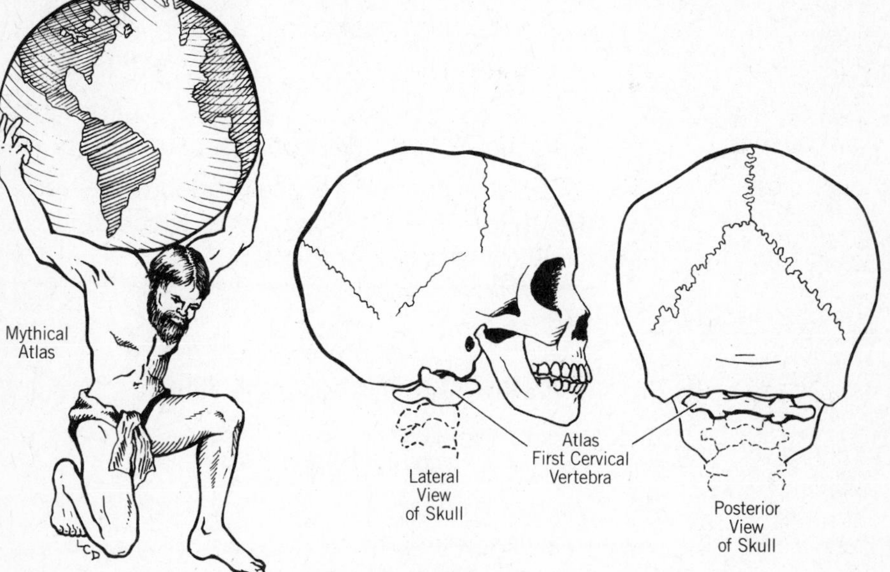

Figure 4.3. THE STORY OF ATLAS

471

The second cervical vertebra is colorfully named the ________ ("axle," frame 412). Inferior to both the ________ (first cervical vertebra) and the skull, it acts as the ________ or central turning point about which these two structures can pivot.

axis
atlas
axis (axle)

472

Look at the following roots, both meaning "tooth":

dens (dens or denz)
odont

Recall that ________, the suffix in *cuboid* (frame 376), means "like" or "resembling." If we use the shorter root, we have simply ________ as "tooth." But if we use the longer root, then ________/________ indicates a "toothlike" condition.

-oid
dens
odont/oid
(ō don' toid)

473

A *process* is a projection, as from the surface of a bone. The ________ ("tooth") or ________* ("toothlike projection") on the superior surface of the ________ (second cervical vertebra) serves as the actual turning point upon which both the skull and atlas pivot (Fig. 4.4).

dens
odontoid process
axis

474

________ ("tooth") is only one of many roots that can take *-oid* as a suffix:

glen "socket"
xyph or *xiph* "sword"
mast "breast"
sphen "wedge"
corac "crow, raven"
ethm "sieve"
styl "stake, pole, pillar"

Odont

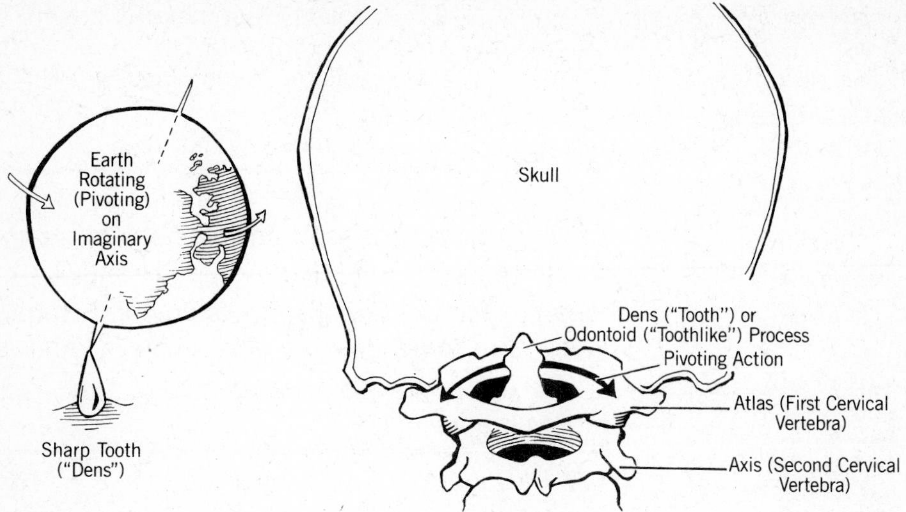

Figure 4.4. THE AXIS

coron	________ "crown" (Unit 1, frame 149) *hy* "the letter U" *pteryg* "wing"

475

Use the information provided in the preceding frame to name each of the things described below:

mast/oid (mas′ toid)	________/______ process "resembles a breast"
hy/oid (hī′ oid)	________/______ bone "resembles the letter U"
sphen/oid (sfē′ noid)	________/______ bone "wedgelike"
ethm/oid (eth′ moid)	________/______ bone "sievelike"
corac/oid (kôr′ ə koid)	________/______ process "resembles a crow"
xyph/oid (xiph/oid) (zif′ oid)	________/______ process "swordlike"
styl/oid (stī′ loid)	________/______ process "resembles a pole or stake"

coron/oid (kôr′ ə noid)	______/_____ fossa "resembles a crown"
glen/oid (glen′ oid, glē′ noid)	______/_____ cavity "resembles a socket"
pteryg/oid (ter′ i goid)	______/_____ process "winglike"

---

tempor stern	**476** *Tempor/al* (tem′ pə rəl) translates as "referring to a temple," where ________, the root, means "temple." *Stern/um* (stûr′ nəm) translates as "presence of the chest," where ________, the root, means "chest," just like *thorac* (frame 100).
tempor/al	**477** The two __________/____ bones form most of the "temples," the flattened regions on each side of the forehead. Perhaps some ancient observer noted that this bone forms the flat side wall of the skull on both right and left, like a "temple" that houses the brain (Fig. 4.5).
temporal mastoid styloid sternum xyphoid (xiphoid)	**478** The ____________ ("temple") bone has both a ____________ ("breastlike") and a ____________ ("stakelike") process projecting downward from it. Likewise the ____________ or "breast bone," located in the middle of the front of the "chest," has a ____________ process projecting downward from it "like a sword" drawn from its sheath (Fig. 4.5)!
hyoid temporal sternum	**479** The ________ bone is an isolated "U-shaped" bone in the neck. It lies inferior to the ____________ ("temple") bone of the skull, but superior to the ____________ ("breast bone" or "chest" bone). (See Fig. 4.5.)

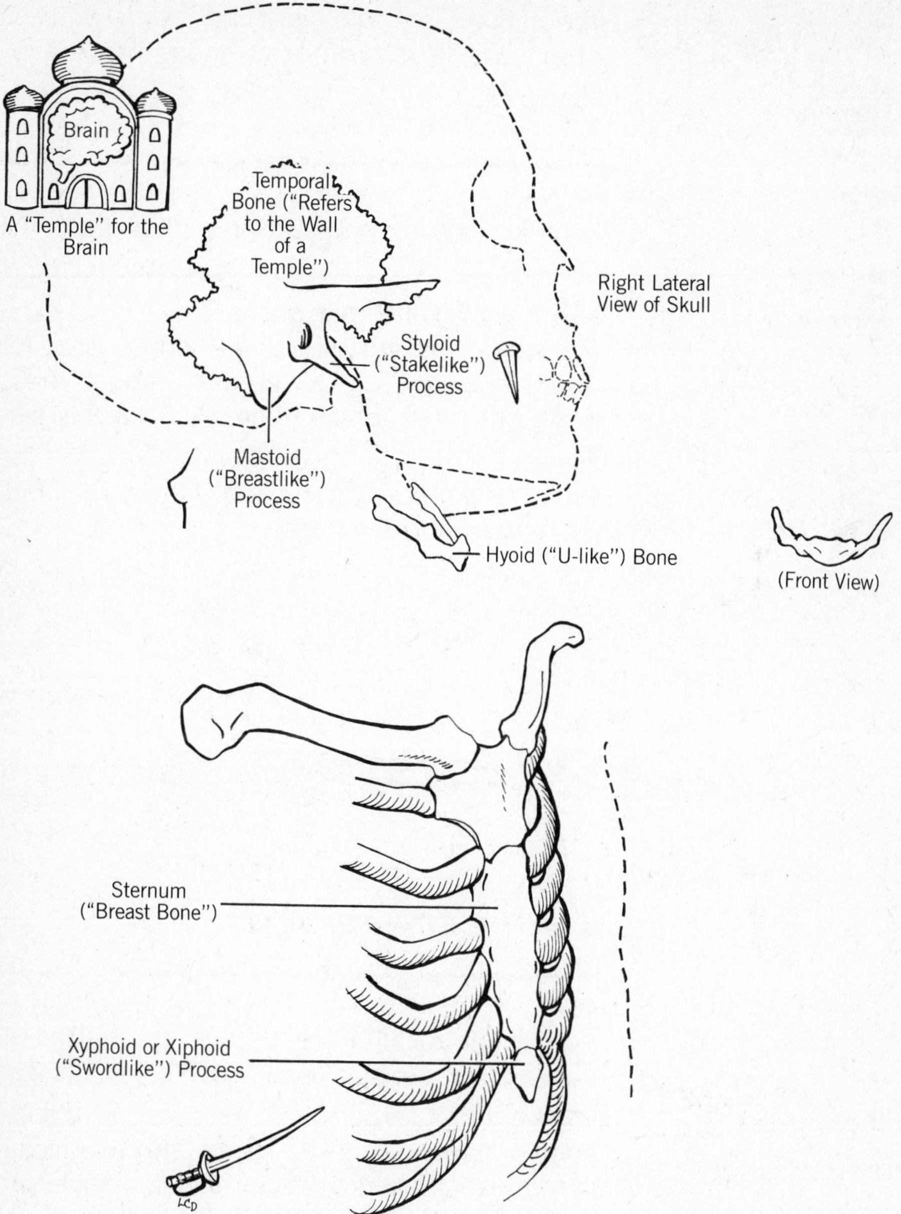

Figure 4.5. TEMPORAL BONE, STERNUM, AND HYOID

ethm

480

Recall from frame 474 that ________ is the root for "sieve." *Cribr* is another root for "sieve," and it often takes *i* as a combining

ethm/oid
cribr/i/form
(krib′ ri fôrm)

vowel. Form is a suffix for either "form" or "like." There are thus two terms meaning "sieve-like": ______/_____ and ______/__/______.

cribriform
ethmoid
cranial

481
Examine Figure 4.6. Observe that both the ______________ ("sievelike") *plate* and much of the rest of the ______________ ("sieve-resembling") *bone* are indeed shot full of holes, quite "like" a "sieve"! Through these holes pass the nerves of smell, since this particular ______________ ("pertaining to the skull," *Word-Building* section, frame 32) bone lies posterior to the nose!

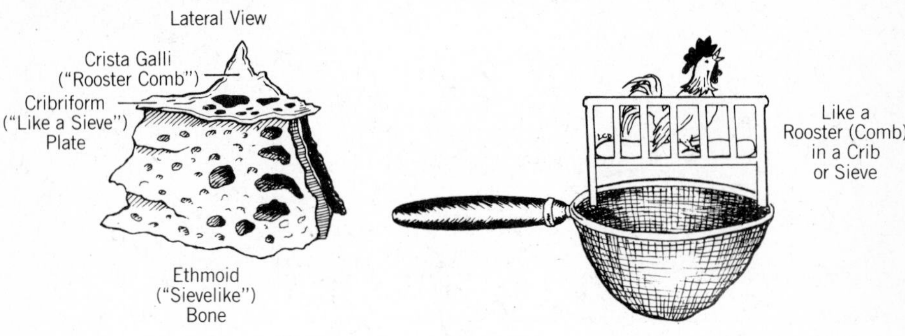

Figure 4.6. THE ETHMOID "SIEVE"

crista
mitochondrion
crista galli

482
You might recall that ______________ (Unit 2, frame 251) means "comb" or "crest." It was used with ______________ ("presence of thread granule," frame 249) to indicate the tiny shelflike projections that resemble the teeth of a hair "comb." Now, however, we are concerned with the *comb* of a *rooster*, the thick red fleshy projection on top of the fowl's head! If *galli* (gal′ ī, gäl′ ē) means "cock" or "rooster," then ______________* means "comb of a rooster"!

crista galli cribriform	**483** A glance at Figure 4.6 reveals that the ______________* ("cock's comb") does indeed project upward from the surface of the ______________ ("sievelike") plate of the ethmoid bone, much like the red fleshy *comb* of an immature rooster lying in its shallow *crib*!
Cribr -form	**484** __________ ("sieve") is not the only root that commonly takes connecting vowel *i* and combines with ________ ("form" or "like"). Another example is *pis*, from the Latin for "pea."
pis/i/form (pī′ si fôrm)	**485** The ______/__/________ bone has the rounded "form" of a single "pea" removed from its pod!
cribriform ethmoid pisiform	**486** The ______________ ("sievelike") *plate* is a thin horizontal portion of the ______________ ("sievelike") *bone* in the skull. But the ______________ bone is a small "pea-shaped" structure in the human wrist.
scapul/a (skap′ yə lə)	**487** *Scapul* means "shoulder blade," so that ____________/__ means "presence of the shoulder blade," where *-a* is the "presence of" suffix.
scapula pisiform appendicular	**488** The ______________ ("shoulder blade presence"), like the ______________ ("pea-formed") bone, is part of the ______________ (axial/appendicular) skeleton.
corac/oid	**489** A glance back at frame 475 reveals that __________/______ denotes resemblance to

glen/oid acromi/on (a krō′ mē on)	a raven or crow, while ______/______ denotes resemblance to a socket. *Acromi* is a root for "shoulder tip" such that ______/______ is "presence of the shoulder tip" just as *diffusion* (frame 295) is "presence of scattering."

---

 acromion glenoid coracoid	**490** The ______________ ("shoulder tip") *process* of the scapula is somewhat like the wingtip of a crow. The ______________ *cavity* is a shallow "socket"-like depression on the lateral edge of the same bone, like a small dent in a bird's breast. And the ______ ________ *process* of the shoulder blade is named for its resemblance to the thick stubby beak of a crow or raven (Fig. 4.7).

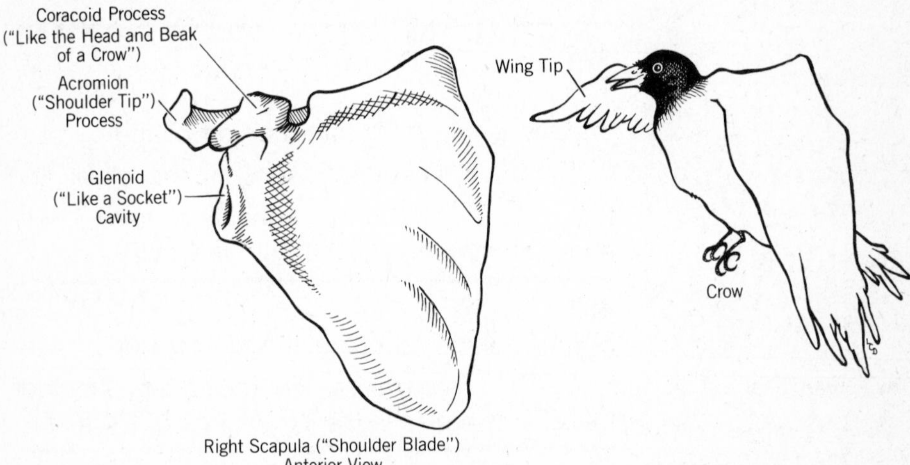

Figure 4.7. ***CORACOID VERSUS CROW***

---

 scapula	**491** Much of a bird can indeed be visualized on the ______________ ("shoulder blade") to make a really good analogy! After all, a crow says "Caw! Caw!," which sounds much like "Corac! Corac!"

492

Seeing some of these analogies certainly requires good imagination and an open mind on your part! But this is what is necessary if you are to grasp the intent of the early scholars and really *understand* the names they first gave to body parts and processes! For example the __________/______ (frame 475) bone has a main central portion or *body* that bears a "resemblance" to a "wedge," like the short stubby wooden wedge used to prop open a door. But the entire bone actually appears more like a bird, bat, or butterfly in flight, since it has both greater and lesser "wings" and ____________/______ ("winglike," frame 475) processes (Fig. 4.8).

sphen/oid

pteryg/oid

493

Sell is Latin for "saddle," and *turcic* stands for "Turkish," as in the country of Turkey. Both roots use ____ as their "presence of" suffix, just as *scapul* (frame 487) does.

-a

494

In what must be one of the most unusual analogies in all of ______________ ("bony," frame 422) anatomy, the saddle-shaped depression in the middle of the top of the _______ ________ ("wedgelike") bone has been named the ________/__ ____________/__ ("presence of a Turkish saddle;" two words). This depression apparently resembles the fancy saddles of the country in question (Fig. 4.8)!

osseous

sphenoid

sell/a turcic/a (sel′ ə; tûr′ si kə)

495

The __________________________* or "Turkish saddle present" on the superior surface of the sphenoid bone actually houses the *pituitary* (pi tyoo′ i terē) gland. But going back to our earlier analogy, this depression is like a fancy saddle on the back of a bat in flight,

sella turcica

Dorsal Posterior View of Sphenoid ("Wedgelike") Bone

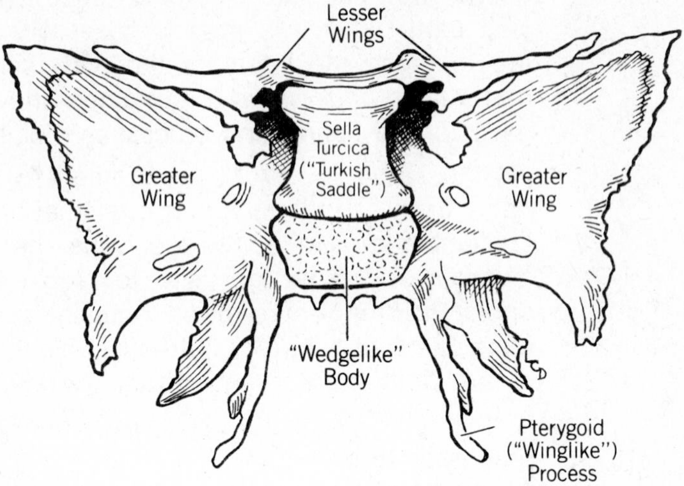

Lesser Wings
Sella Turcica ("Turkish Saddle")
Greater Wing
Greater Wing
"Wedgelike" Body
Pterygoid ("Winglike") Process

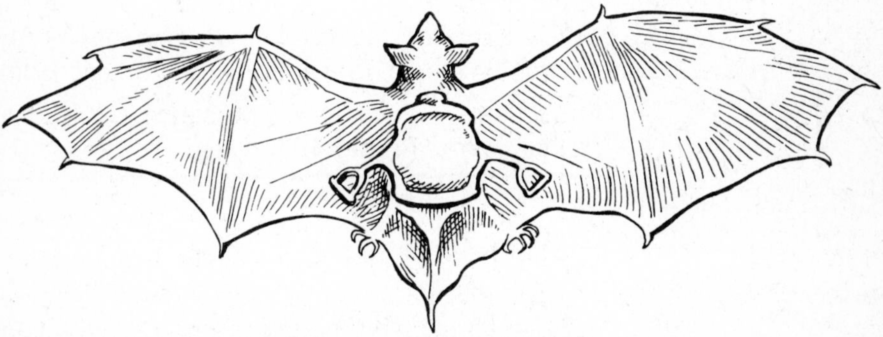

Bat in Flight (Top View) with Saddle

Lateral View
Sella Turcica
Turkish Saddle

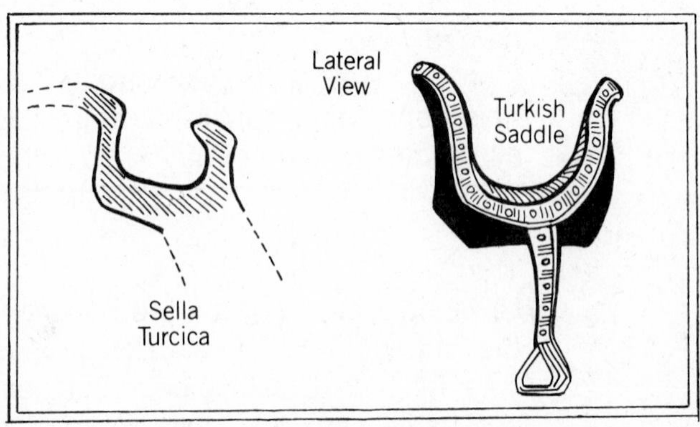

Figure 4.8. BONES AND BATS

Answer	Frame
pterygoid	with the ________________ ("wing-resembling") processes extending downward like hairy flapping legs (Fig. 4.8)!
foss/a (fos′ ə)	**496** If *foss* means "trench, ditch, or depression," then ________/__ is a term for "presence of a depression," where *-a* is the appropriate suffix.
process fossa	**497** While a ______________ (frame 473) represents a bony *projection*, a __________ must represent a bony *depression*, since these two terms are exactly opposite in meaning.
sella turcica fossa	**498** The __________________________* is a saddle-shaped __________ ("depression") on the superior surface of the sphenoid bone.
glenoid scapula	**499** The ______________ ("socketlike," frame 490) *cavity* is another example of a fossa, this one present on the lateral aspect of the ______________ ("shoulder blade").
-us	**500** *Humer* means "shoulder" and takes _____, the same ending found in *canaliculus* (frame 437), as its "presence of" suffix.
Humer/us (hyo͞o′ mər əs) proximal fossa scapula	**501** __________/____ is literally translated from the Latin as "presence of the shoulder." Perhaps this is so because the upper ______________ ("near," frame 166) end or "head" of this bone inserts into the glenoid __________ ("depression, cavity") of the __________ ("shoulder blade") (Fig. 4.9).
humerus	**502** The ______________ is the upper arm bone,

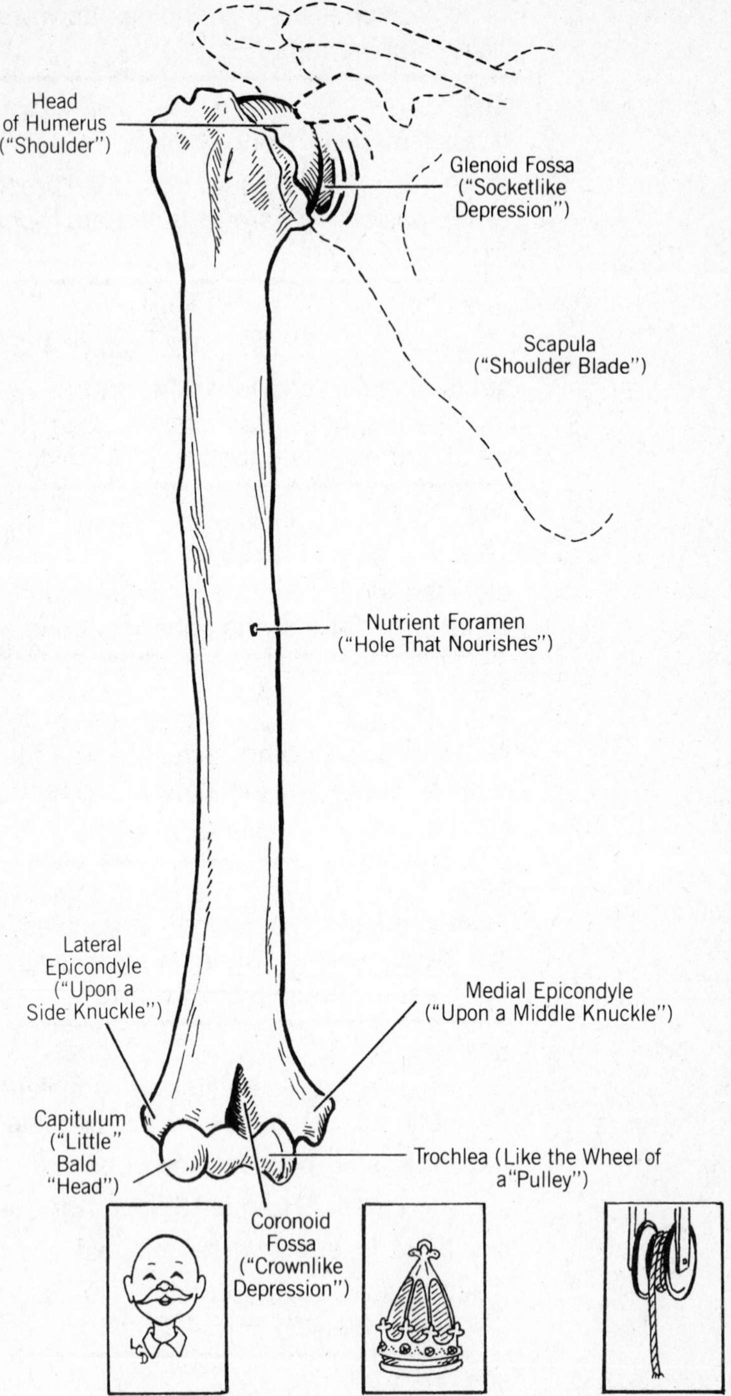

Figure 4.9. RIGHT HUMERUS AT THE SHOULDER (ANTERIOR VIEW)

and as you can see from Figure 4.9, its "head" forms the *shoulder joint* with the glenoid fossa. Hence its name of "shoulder."

503

crown

Recall that *coron* (frame 474) is the root for "________."

504

coronoid

Returning a final time to frame 475, we can say that ________ means "resembling a crown."

505

coronoid fossa

distal

The ________________* is the "crown-shaped depression present" on the anterior surface of the humerus, at the ________ ("distant," frame 166) extremity of the bone (Fig. 4.9).

506

humerus

epi/condyl/e (ep i kon′ dīl)

epi-

The distal end of the ________ (upper arm bone) also is associated with a number of different *condyles* (kon′ dīlz). If *condyl/e* means "presence of a knuckle," then ____/ ________/__ means "presence upon a knuckle," where ______, the prefix in *epiphysis* (frame 452), means "upon."

507

lateral

epicondyle

Figure 4.9 demonstrates both a ________ ("toward the side") *epicondyle* and a *medial* ________________ ("presence upon a knuckle") at the lower end of the humerus.

508

condyle

By definition each *epicondyle* must rest upon a ________ (term for "knuckle").

509

trochle/a (trok′ lē ə)

If *trochle* is a root for "pulley," then ______ ______/__ is a term meaning "presence of a pulley," where the "presence of" suffix is the same as that found with *scapula* (frame 487).

---

trochlea

510
The ______________ is a condyle on the distal end of the humerus that looks much like the grooved wheel or spool of a "pulley" (Fig. 4.9).

---

epicondyle

511
The medial ______________ lies "upon the knuckle" of the trochlea. You can feel it with your fingertips as a prominent bump on the medial aspect of the elbow. It is often referred to as the "funny bone."

---

head
little head

512
Capit, like *cephal* (frame 135), means "________." And *capitul* must consequently mean "______________,"* in much the same way that *articul* (frame 455) means "little joint."

Capitul/um
(ka pit′ yə ləm)

513
______________/____ is the proper anatomical term denoting the "presence of a little head," where the suffix is the same as that in *periosteum* (frame 449).

---

capitulum

514
The ______________ is a rounded knuckle or condyle at the lower extremity of the humerus, and it does indeed resemble a "little" bald "head" (Fig. 4.9)!

-ent

515
A *foramen* (fō rā′ mən) is a "hole" or "passage." And *nutri* means "suckle, nurse, or nourish." According to Table 8 (frame 55, *Word-Building* section) and frame 275, ________ is a suffix for "one that."

---

nutri/ent
(nyo͞o′ trē ənt)

516
Thus ________/______ means "one that

foramen	nourishes." A ____________ ("hole") may provide a point of entry for blood vessels nourishing the interior of a bone.
nutrient foramen medullary	**517** For example, the humerus has a ____________ ____________* ("hole that nourishes") through which blood vessels feed into the ____________ ("middle" or "marrow," frame 446) cavity (Fig. 4.9).
process fossa condyle epicondyle foramen osseous	**518** Whether we are discussing a ____________ (bony "projection"), ____________ ("depression"), ____________ ("knuckle"), ____________ ____________ ("upon knuckle"), or a ____________ ____________ ("hole"), the interesting analogies could go on and on! Using your own common sense, imagination, and a handy medical dictionary, you can decipher the meanings of many other ____________ ("bony," frame 422) terms you may encounter.

Now do the Self-Test for Unit 4 (page 268 in the Appendix).

UNIT 5
TERMS OF THE MUSCLES AND MOVEMENT

muscul	**519** Each of the six different roots below mean *musc* "mouse" or "muscle" __________ "little mouse" (muscle), as *cellul* (frame 185) means "little chamber" *my* "muscle" *myos* "muscle" *mys* "muscle" *sarc* "flesh" (muscle)
intra- -ar	**520** *Neur/o* indicates "nerve" and __________ (as in *intracellular*, frame 189) is a prefix for "within." *Muscul* takes ______, the suffix in *intracellular*, as its "pertaining to" ending.
Muscul/ar muscul	**521** __________/____ could literally be interpreted as "pertaining to a little mouse"! Perhaps some ancient scholar compared a small muscle to a little mouse running across the dissection table! Isn't it ironic that the muscles, those symbols of power and strength, should have the root __________ ("little mouse") applied to them?
	522 This "little mouse" root is commonly used with other word parts to describe various aspects of muscle. For example, logic tells us that

Table 5.1 GENERAL TERMS OF MUSCLES AND MOVEMENTS

abduction	flexion	myosin
abductor	flexor	neuromuscular
actin	fusiform	perimysium
adduction	intramuscular	sarcolemma
adductor	isometric	sarcomere
endomysium	isotonic	sarcoplasm
epimysium	ligament	sarcoplasmic reticulum
extension	muscular	tendon
extensor	myofibril	
fascicle	myofilament	

intra/muscul/ar

neur/o/muscul/ar (nyoo′ rō mus′ kyo͞o lər)

________/__________/____ "refers to (something) within a muscle," and that ________/__/__________/____ must "pertain to both nerve and muscle" together.

---

intramuscular

523

A nurse may give a patient an ______________________ ("within muscle") injection when slow continuous absorption of a drug into the bloodstream is desirable.

---

neuromuscular

524

An injected drug may act by blocking the transmission of messages across the ______________________ ("nerve-muscle") junction.

-um

525

Mys is another root in frame 519 which starts with "m" and means "muscle." It takes *i* as its combining vowel and ______, the suffix in *epithelium* (frame 117), *endosteum* (frame 447), and *periosteum* (frame 449), as its "presence of" ending.

---

mys/i/um (miz′ ē əm)

526

Consequently ______/__/____ is a term denoting "presence of a muscle." Using each of the three different prefixes found within the

epi/mys/i/um (ep i miz' ē əm) peri/mys/i/um (per i miz' ē əm) endo/mys/i/um (en dō miz ē əm)	terms of frame 525, go ahead and build new terms meaning: _____/_____ /__/____ "presence upon muscle" _____/_____ /__/____ "presence around muscle" _____/_____ /__/____ "presence within muscle"
fascia	**527** Recall that __________ (frame 368) is a milky fibrous connective "sheet" enveloping and subdividing many of the body organs.
Epimysium	**528** ______________ is the layer of fascia that lies "upon" the surface of the entire "muscle" (Fig. 5.1).

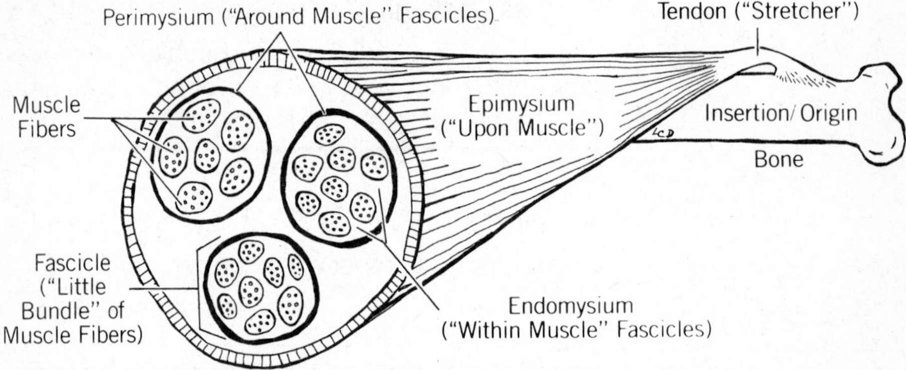

Figure 5.1. FUSIFORM ("SPINDLE-SHAPED") MUSCLE: CROSS-SECTION

Perimysium	**529** ______________ is the layer of fascia that is "present around" isolated bundles of fibers inside the "muscle" (Fig. 5.1).
endomysium	**530** And ______________ is the fascia "present within" the bundles of individual "muscle" fibers (Fig. 5.1).

-le

fascic/le (fas′ i kəl)

531
Fascic like fasci (frame 367) is a root for "band" or "sheet," and ______, the suffix in *vesicle* (frame 240), means "little." Use this information to build __________/____, a term meaning "little bundle."

perimysium

fascicles

532
Inside of a muscle, ________________ is the fascia around the bundles of muscle fibers, actually forming the ________________ ("small bundles") (Fig. 5.1).

endomysium

fascicle

533
And ________________ is the fascia within each small bundle or ______________, separating the adjacent muscle fibers within the bundle (Fig. 5.1).

fus/i/form

534
The muscle pictured in Figure 5.1 is *fusiform* (fyo͞o′ zi fôrm). *Fus* means "spindle." Subdivide *fusiform* just as you did *cribriform* (frame 480): ______/__/______.

fusiform

535
Just as *cribriform* means "having the form of a sieve," ______________ means "having the form of a spindle," that is, wide in the center and tapered at each end.

fusiform

536
A ______________ ("spindle-shaped") muscle has a *tendon* (ten′ dən) at each end. *Tend* means "stretch."

Tend/on

537
_______/_____ is translated as "presence of a stretcher," where the suffix is the same as that in *mitochondrion* (frame 246).

tendon

538
There is normally a __________ ("stretch-

fusiform	er") present at each end of a ________ ________ ("spindlelike") muscle, connecting the muscle to bone.
epimysium	**539** The ________________ (fascia "present upon muscle") extends over the entire external muscle surface and continues out as a tendon at each end, much like the cellophane wrapper that is twisted and narrow at each extremity of a hard piece of red Christmas candy.
tendon	**540** The ____________ ("stretcher") is "stretched" when the muscle contracts and shortens in length, pulling on the ends.
ligament	**541** *Ligament* (lig′ ə mənt) is the Latin root for "band" or "bandage." A ______________ is like a "bandage" of tough fibrous connective tissue that straps together two or more bones and/or cartilages.
Tendons ligaments	**542** ______________ (Tendons/Ligaments) attach muscles to bones, whereas ______________ ______________ (tendons/ligaments) attach bones to each other.
sarc plasm -mere	**543** Return to frame 519. Note that ________ is the root for "flesh," that is, "muscle." It is commonly used with each of the following: lemm ________ "husk" ________ "matter" (frame 191) ________ "segment" (suffix found in frame 228) It takes *o* as its combining vowel.

Sarc/o/lemm/a (sär kō lem' ə)	**544** ______/__/________/__ is the term denoting "presence of a flesh husk," where the suffix is identical to that in *lacuna* (frame 432).
sarcolemma	**545** Just as a tough green fibrous husk covers an ear of corn, the ______________ ("flesh husk") forms a protective membrane for the individual skeletal muscle fiber (Fig. 5.2).

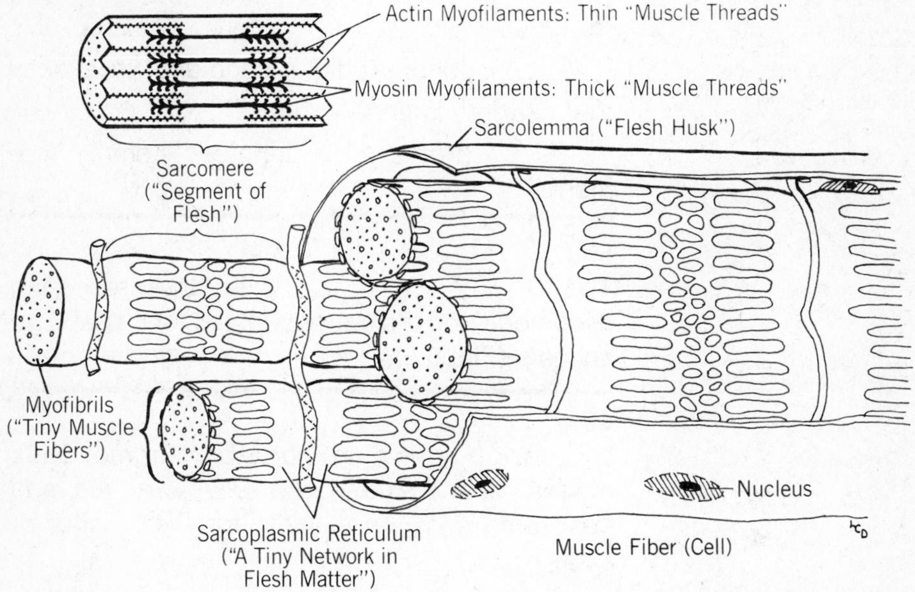

Figure 5.2. CROSS-SECTION OF A SKELETAL MUSCLE FIBER

sarc/o/plasm (sär' kō plaz əm)	**546** Just as *cytoplasm* (frame 194) or "cell matter" occupies much of the cell interior, ______/__/________ or "flesh matter" occupies much of the muscle fiber interior.
sarcoplasmic	**547** And just as the *endoplasmic reticulum* (frame 200) is a "tiny network present within (cell) matter," the ______________

reticulum	______________* is a "tiny network present (in) flesh matter."
sarcoplasmic reticulum	**548** Like the ER, the ______________ ______________* serves as a transport system of many "networks" of channels, this time associated with the muscle fiber (Fig. 5.2).
segment sarc/o/mere (sär' kō mir) centr/o/mere	**549** Observe that *-mere* in frame 543 is the suffix for "______________." Then ______/__/______ denotes "flesh segment" in exactly the same manner that ______/__/______ (frame 228) denotes "central segment."
sarcomere	**550** The ______________ is the repeating "segment" of the muscle fibers or "flesh" of animals (Fig. 5.2).
Fibr fibr/il	**551** ______, a root in *fibroblast* (frame 355), means "fiber." And *-il,* like *-elle, -ole, -ule*, and *-le* (frame 241), is a suffix for "tiny, little, or small." A ______/____ is thus a "tiny fiber."
My my/o/fibr/il (mī' ō fī' bril)	**552** ____ is the third root mentioned in frame 519 which means "muscle." It generally takes *o* as its combining vowel. Thus ____/__/______/____ translates as "tiny muscle fiber."
myofibril	**553** The muscle *fiber* is actually a complete *cell*, while the ______________ ("tiny muscle fiber") is in reality a fiber-shaped ______

Answers	Frames
organelle	________ ("miniature organ," frame 203) within the fiber (Fig. 5.2).
-ent filam/ent	**554** *Filam* means "thread" and it combines with ________, the suffix of *nutrient* (frame 516) to make ________/______ ("one that is a thread").
my/o/filam/ent (mī′ ō fil′ ə mənt)	**555** Just as *myofibril* literally means "tiny muscle fiber," ____/__/__________/______ means "muscle that is a thread."
Myofilaments sarcomere myofibril	**556** ______________________ are actually "threadlike" protein rods present within each ______________ (repeating muscle "segment") of a ______________ ("tiny muscle fiber" organelle) (Fig. 5.2).
microscopic	**557** These ________________ ("referring to examining small things," frame 409) myofilaments are of two different types: *actin* (ak′ tin) and *myosin* (mī′ ə sin).
Myos	**558** Refer back to frame 519 one last time. ________ is the root for "muscle," which combines with *-in* to make *myosin*.
Myos/in	**559** The suffix, *-in*, is generally used in chemistry to indicate "a neutral substance" (neither acid nor base) such as fats or proteins. ________/____ then means "a neutral substance" in "muscle."
	560 *Act* comes from the Latin for "motion." Conse-

act/in	quently ______/____ is a term which translates as "a neutral substance" in "motion."
Myosin protein myofilaments sarcomere	**561** ____________ ("neutral substance" in "muscle") is a ______________ ("first" chemical, frame 322) that occurs in stationary thick ____ ____________________ ("muscle-threads") located in the middle of each __________ ________ ("flesh segment") (Fig. 5.2).
Actin myofilaments sarcomere	**562** __________ ("neutral substance" in "motion") is a protein that occurs in nonstationary thin _______________________ ("muscle-threads") located at the edges of each ______ ____________ ("muscle segment") (Fig. 5.2).
thin actin	**563** During muscle contraction, it is the ________ ____________* (thin actin/thick myosin) myofilaments that slide inward toward the center of the sarcomere. Hence the root *act*, which means "motion," denotes the inward motion of these structures during contraction and their outward motion during relaxation.
physiological muscular	**564** *Actin* is named for its _________________ ________ (anatomical/physiological) property of sliding inward-outward motion. Other ________________ ("referring to little mouse," frame 521) terms also relate to function.
iso- ton/ic	**565** For example, recall from Unit 2 (frame 287) that ________ is a prefix meaning "same, equal, or constant," and that ______/____ (frame 286) is a term which translates as "pertaining to strength or tension." *Metr* is Latin for "length."

Iso/ton/ic

iso/metr/ic
(ī sō met′ rik)

566
______/______/____ "refers to constant tension," while ______/________/____ "refers to constant length."

isotonic

567
An ______________ (isotonic/isometric) contraction is one in which the muscle shortens in length but maintains a *constant* degree of *tension*.

isometric

568
An ________________ (isotonic/isometric) contraction is one of *constant length*. The muscle builds tension but is not allowed to shorten.

isotonic

-ion

-or

569
The ______________ (isotonic/isometric) contractions of various skeletal muscles lead to different types of body movements. These diverse movements are described by different roots, followed by the same suffix, ______ ("the act or process of"), as found within *solution* (frame 275). When roots describing these movements are followed by _____ ("one which or one who"), the suffix in *inferior* (frame 141), they are used as general names for muscles themselves.

toward (etc.)

570
To be specific, observe the following roots:

extens "stretching out or straightening out"
flex "bending"
duct "movement"

Ab- is a prefix meaning "away from," while *ad-*, its opposite, means "____________."

571
Now employ the information provided within frames 569–570 to build terms with the following meanings:

flex/ion (flek′ shən)	________/________ "the act/process of bending"
flex/or (flek′ sər)	________/____ "one which bends"
extens/ion	________/______ "the act/process of straightening"
extens/or (eks ten′ sər)	________/____ "one which straightens"
ad/duct/ion (a duk′ shən)	____/________/______ "the act/process of moving (something) toward"
ad/duct/or (a duk′ tər)	____/________/____ "one which moves (something) toward"
ab/duct/ion (ab duk′ shən)	____/________/______ "the act/process of moving (something) away from"
ab/duct/or (ab duk′ tər)	____/________/____ "one which moves (something) away from"

572

We can thus conclude that a muscle should be given the general name of ____________ (extensor/flexor) if it causes movement which "straightens out" or increases the angle between two bones at a joint. And ____________ (extension/flexion) is the term that describes this straightening act.

Answers: extensor; extension

573

Conversely, a muscle should be given the classification of ____________ if it causes motion which "bends" a body limb or otherwise decreases the angle between two bones at a joint. And ____________ is the term that describes this bending act.

Answers: flexor; flexion

574

In a similar manner, an ____________ (adductor/abductor) is a muscle that moves a limb "away from" the main body trunk. ____________ (Adduction/Abduction) is the term that describes this process of moving away from the trunk.

Answers: abductor; Abduction

adductor

adduction

575
Conversely, an ______________ is a muscle that moves a limb "toward" the main body trunk. And ______________ describes its general mode of action.

-or

-ion

576
You should be able to see by now that you can give names to muscles by adding a suffix like ______ ("one which" or "one who") to different roots. And it should be obvious that you can build a term indicating that an "act or process of" doing something occurred simply by attaching the suffix ________ to the appropriate root.

muscular

577
If you have access to a good dictionary, you should be capable of deciphering the meanings of many other general ______________ ("little mouse") terms that you may encounter during your studies.

Table 5.2 TERMS OF SELECTED MUSCLES AND ASSOCIATED STRUCTURES

abdominis	intercostal
Achilles' tendon	masseter
biceps brachii	oblique
biceps femoris	orbicular
buccinator	pectoralis major
clavicle	quadriceps femoris
costal	rectus abdominis
deltoid	soleus
femoris	sternocleidomastoid
gastrocnemius	tibialis
gluteus	transverse abdominis
gluteus maximus	trapezius
humerus	triceps brachii

578
There are a number of useful features often used in the naming of individual skeletal muscles. One of these criteria is simple geometric

Delt/oid (del′ toid)

Orbicul/ar (ôr bik′ yə lər)

shape. Observe the following list of roots for shapes:

delt "triangle"
orbicul "little orbit or small circle"
trapez "table"

_____/_____ means "resembling a triangle," just as *hyoid* (frame 475) means "resembling a U." _____/_____ translates as "pertaining to a little orbit," where the suffix is identical to that in both *reticular* (frame 357) and *appendicular* (frame 411).

Trapez

-us

humerus

trapez/i/us (tra pē′ zē əs)

579

_____ ("table") commonly takes *i* as its connecting vowel, and often _____, the ending in _____ ("presence of the shoulder," frame 501), serves as its suffix. Consequently _____/__/_____ means "presence of a table."

---

deltoid

abductor

580

The _____ muscle is a large "triangular" muscle forming much of the fleshy shoulder pad. It is an _____ (abductor/adductor) of the arm, acting to draw the arm away from the main body trunk.

---

trapezius

posterior

581

The _____ is a "table"-like muscle "present" on the _____ ("one which is behind," frame 160) aspect of the neck, the upper shoulder, and the upper back. Although somewhat resembling a four-sided table individually, both the muscle on the right and left sides of the body taken together roughly appear to have the shape of a diamond.

Orbicular

582

_____ ("little orbit") muscles form circular rings or *sphincters* (sfingk′ tərz) located around various body openings, such as

oral	those of the ________ ("mouth," frame 104) cavity and the eye.
	583 Here are some roots for *locations*: *femor* "thigh" *tibi* "shin bone" *brachi* "arm" *pector* "breast" or "chest" *glute* "buttock" *cost* "rib" *gastrocnemi* "calf" *sole* "sole of the foot" or "sandal"
abdomin	______________ "abdomen" (trunk midsection), frame 89
	584 The roots in the preceding frame make use of various suffixes when involved in the naming of specific muscles. For example, we have
femor/is (fem′ ər is)	both __________/____ ("presence of the
abdomin/is (ab dom′ i nis)	thigh") and ______________/____ ("presence of the abdomen") using the suffix of *cutis* (frame 386).
	585
Cost/al (kos′ təl)	________/____ ("referring to the ribs") takes the same suffix found in *parietal* (frame 82).
inter-	Recall that __________, the prefix in *interphase* (frame 344), means "between." Thus
inter/cost/al (in tər kos′ təl)	__________/________/____ translates as "referring to (something) between the ribs."
	586
intercostal	The external and internal ________________ ______ ("between the ribs") muscles help to change the size of the chest cage during breathing.
	587 Like *-al*, the suffix *-alis* also means "pertaining
tibi/alis (tib ē ā′ lis)	or referring to," as in ________/________

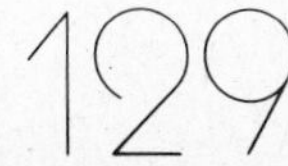

pector/alis
(pek tə rā′ lis)

("pertaining to the shin bone") and _____ _____/_____ ("referring to the chest or breast").

---

tibialis

588
The __________ *anterior* muscle by definition is located "in front of the shin bone" in the lower leg.

---

glute/us (glo͞o′ tē əs)
gastrocnemi/us
(gas′ trək nē′ mē əs)
sole/us (sō′ lē əs)

589
Remember that the suffix in *nucleus* (frame 207) means "presence of." Consequently, referring back to frame 583, we construct _______/___ ("presence of the buttocks"), _______________/___ ("presence of the calf"), and finally _____/___ ("presence of the sole").

---

gastrocnemius
soleus
flex

590
The ________________ is the main muscle "present" in the "calf," but the ________ is also "present" in the lower leg to help _____ ("bend," frame 570) the foot such that the toes dip downward toward the "sole."

---

bi-
tri-
bi/ceps (bī′ seps)
tri/ceps (trī′ seps)

591
Another criterion for muscle nomenclature is the number of *ceps* ("heads" or divisions) in a muscle. A *bicycle* has *two* wheels. So _____, like *di-*, means "two." And ______ (frame 316) means "three." Then _____/_____ means "two heads" and _____/_____ means "three heads."

---

biceps brachii
(bī′ seps brā′ kē ī)

592
We can combine these terms for number of muscle heads with terms for muscle location. For example, the ____________ _____* is a "two-headed" muscle in the

upper "arm," where the root for "arm" in frame 583 has had an additional "i" added to it for easier pronunciation.

---

triceps brachii

593
Similarly the ______________________________*
is a "three-headed" muscle in the upper "arm."

Flex

triceps brachii

extend

594
These two arm muscles have opposite or antagonistic actions. Whereas the *biceps brachii* acts to ________ (extend/flex) the lower arm by "bending" it at the elbow, the ________ ______________________* ("three-headed arm" muscle) acts to ____________ (extend/flex) the lower arm by "straightening" it at the elbow.

---

femoris

biceps femoris

595
Recall from frame 584 that ____________ means "presence of the thigh." It is logical to give the name __________________________* to a muscle with "two heads present" on the back of the "thigh."

---

four

quadri/ceps
(kwäd′ ri seps)

596
Quadri- is a prefix for "________" (one/two/three/four). Consequently, the ____________/ ________ ("four-headed") *femoris* is a group of "four" anterior muscles "present on the thigh" that together act to extend the lower leg.

---

quadriceps femoris

biceps femoris

597
The ___________________________________*
("four-headed thigh" muscle group) is antagonistic to the ____________________________*
("two-headed thigh" muscle).

598
A fourth muscle characteristic used in naming is relative muscle *size*. For example we would

gluteus maximus	expect the ___________________* (*gluteus maximus/gluteus medius/gluteus minimus*) to be the largest muscle that is "present" in the "buttocks" or "rump." This is because it is the one of "maximum" size!
pectoralis major	**599** It is likewise reasonable to suppose that the ___________________* (*pectoralis minor/pectoralis major*) is the larger muscle of higher rank or importance "present" in the "breast or chest" region.
transverse	**600** A fifth criterion for muscle naming concerns the *direction of muscle fibers*. Look at the following: *rect* "vertical;" uses suffix *-us* ___________ "presence of a turning across" (frame 132) *obliqu* "slanted;" often uses suffix *-e*
Rect/us obliqu/e (ō blēk′)	**601** _______/____ indicates the "presence of vertical" muscle fibers, whereas ________/__ describes the "presence of slanted" fibers within a muscle.
abdominis	**602** Remember from frame 594 that ___________ means "presence of the abdomen."
oblique rectus abdominis	**603** Now use the information of frames 600–602 to build the proper anatomical names for the muscles described in this narration: "The *internal* and *external* ___________ muscles have 'slanted' fibers 'present' on the sides of the lower body trunk. The ___________________* is a strap-like muscle with 'vertical' fibers 'present' on the anterior wall of the 'abdomen.'

flexor	It is the main __________ ('bender,' frame 571) of the trunk and is often dubbed the *sit-ups* muscle.
transverse abdominis	The ______________________________* is a deep horizontal muscle 'present' in the lateral wall of the 'abdomen.' Its fibers 'turn' and pass partially 'across' the front of the abdominal wall to form a *living girdle* of muscle tissue."
-or	**604** A sixth criterion for muscle nomenclature is *specific muscle function*. Observe these two roots: *masset* "chew;" uses *-er* ("a thing that") as a suffix *buccinat* "trumpet;" uses ____, the suffix in *extensor* (frame 571)
Masset/er (ma sē′ tər) buccinat/or (buk′ si nā tər)	**605** __________/____ translates as "a thing that chews," while __________/____ literally means "one that trumpets."
masseter	**606** The __________ ("chewer") helps to lift the lower jaw during the chewing process.
buccinator bucc	**607** The __________ ("trumpeter") compresses the wall of the cheek during the blowing of a horn or trumpet. Recall that __________ (frame 102) is the root for "cheek."
osseous tendons	**608** A seventh characteristic useful for naming is *points of muscle attachment*. Muscles can be named by the __________ ("bony," frame 422) attachments of their __________ ("stretchers," frame 537).

stern
stern
sternum

609
For example ________ (frame 476), like *thorac* (frame 100) and *pector* (frame 583) means either "breast" or "chest." Thus ________/o represents the root and combining vowel for indicating tendons which attach muscles to the ________ ("breast bone," frame 476).

-le
cuticle
fascicle

610
Both *cleid* and *clavic* mean "key." The latter root combines with ____, the suffix in *vesicle* (frame 240), ________ ("little skin," frame 389), and ________ ("little bundle," frame 531).

clavic/le (klav′ i kəl)

611
Therefore ________/____ denotes a "little key."

clavicle
medial/mesial
lateral
scapula

612
The ________ or *collar bone* is a "small" bone lying horizontally at the base of the neck, right at the level of a shirt collar. It looks somewhat like a plain "key." Its ________ ("pertaining to the middle," frame 154) extremity forms a joint with the *sternum*, while its ________ ("referring to the side," frame 157) end joins with the ________ ("shoulder blade," frame 487) (Fig. 5.3).

Cleid

613
________, the first root for "key" given in frame 610, takes the combining vowel *o* when it is used to indicate tendons attaching to the *clavicle*.

temporal

614
Remember from frame 478 that the ________ ("temple") bone of the skull has a

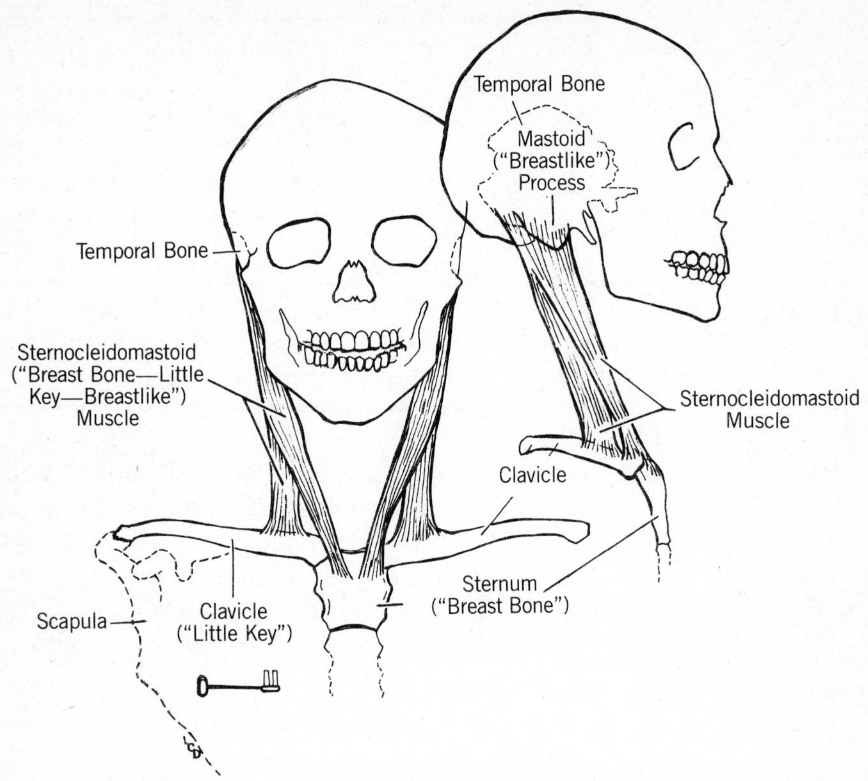

Figure 5.3. THE STERNOCLEIDOMASTOID

mast/oid	_________/_______ ("breast-resembling") process.
stern/o/cleid/o/ mast/oid (stûr′ nō klī′ dō mas′ toid)	**615** Finally putting the facts in frames 609, 613, and 614 together, you can construct ___________/ __/___________/__/__________/______, a single long term that represents the *breast bone, collar bone*, and the "breastlike" process of the temple.
sternocleidomastoid	**616** The ______________________________ muscle originates from the *sternum* and the *clavicle*. Slanting upward and backward along the side of the neck, it inserts on the *mastoid* process of the temporal bone (Fig. 5.3).

sternocleidomastoid

cervical

vertebral

617
The ______________________ (sternum-clavicle-mastoid process) is sometimes called the "prayer" muscle. When both the right and left muscles act together they flex the ______________ ("pertaining to the neck," frame 468) portion of the ______________ ("jointed backbone," frame 106) column, bowing the head downward and forward toward the chest as if in "prayer."

Achilles

618
An extremely colorful criterion for naming body structures is *association with mythological characters*. For example, *Achilles* (ə kil′ ēz) was a famous warrior in Greek mythology. His mother held him by the heels and dipped him into the River Styx, the River of Immortality, at an early age. Thus ______________ was invulnerable in battle except for his heels, which had not touched the magic water. During the Trojan War an arrow was supposedly shot into Achilles' unprotected heel, thereby killing him!

Achilles' tendon

gastrocnemius

619
Feel the prominent ______________________* (mythological Greek warrior + "presence of a stretcher," frame 537) forming a broad ridge at the back of your heel. Your fingers can trace much of its length, from the heel bone at the bottom to the ______________________ (major "calf" muscle "present," frame 590) at the top. This is the site where the fatal arrow lodged!

shape

620
We have just scratched the surface of muscle nomenclature. But you can list at least eight different criteria for naming muscles and associated structures:

a ______________________

location	b ______________________
number of heads	c ______________________
size	d ______________________
direction of fibers	e ______________________
specific function	f ______________________
points of attachment	g ______________________
association with mythological characters	h ______________________
(All of the above in any order.)	

Now do the Self-Test for Unit 5 (page 271 in the Appendix).

UNIT 6
TERMS OF THE NERVOUS SYSTEM

nerv/ous neur/al	**621** *Nerv* comes from Latin while *neur* derives from Greek. Both of them refer to "nerve," a whitish cord of tissue that conducts information about the environment from one part of the body to another. The first root takes the ending of *serous* (frame 412), while the second joins with the "pertaining to" suffix in *epithelial* (frame 381). Thus ______/_____ and ______/____ both "refer to nerve."
nervous neural	**622** You have probably heard of the __________ (nervous/neural) *system*, much of which begins as a hollow __________ (nervous/neural) *tube*. This tube eventually matures to form the brain, brainstem, spinal cord, and *nerves*, which enter and leave these structures.
encephal encephalon (en sef′ ə lon)	**623** The brain is located "within the head." Recall that __________ (frame 52) is the root for "within head" or "brain," and that __________ means "presence of the brain."
encephalon	**624** The various regions of the __________ ("brain presence") can be distin-

Table 6.1 TERMS OF GROSS BRAIN STRUCTURE

arachnoid mater	gyri	nervous
basal ganglia	gyrus	neural
cerebellum	hypophysis	optic chiasm
cerebral	hypothalamus	peduncle
cerebral cortex	intermediate mass	pia mater
cerebrospinal	mammillary	pituitary
cerebrum	maters	pons
colliculi	medulla oblongata	spinal
colliculus	meninges	subarachnoid
corpora quadrigemina	mesencephalon	sulci
diencephalon	metencephalon	sulcus
dura mater	myelencephalon	telencephalon
encephalon		thalamus
ganglion		ventricle

Answers	Frame
tel- telencephalon (tel′ ən sef′ ə lon)	guished simply by the use of different prefixes. For example, you learned way back in frame 53 that ________ is a prefix for "end" and that the ________________ is the region "present" on the front "end" of the "brain."
middle two/double di/encephal/on (dī′ ən sef′ ə lon) mes/encephal/on (mez′ en sef′ ə lon) met/encephal/on myel/encephal/on (mī əl en sef′ ə lon)	**625** *Mes* (frame 153) is a root meaning "____________." *Di-* (frame 310) like *bi-* (frame 591) means "________________." *Met* means "after," and myel is a root for "spinal cord." Use this information to name the brain regions described: ____/______________/____ the region consisting of "two" major "brain" areas; ______/______________/____ the "middle brain" region; ________/______________/____ the "brain" region occurring just "after" the middle brain; __________/______________/____ the lowest region of the "brain;" which merges with the "spinal cord" (Fig. 6.1).

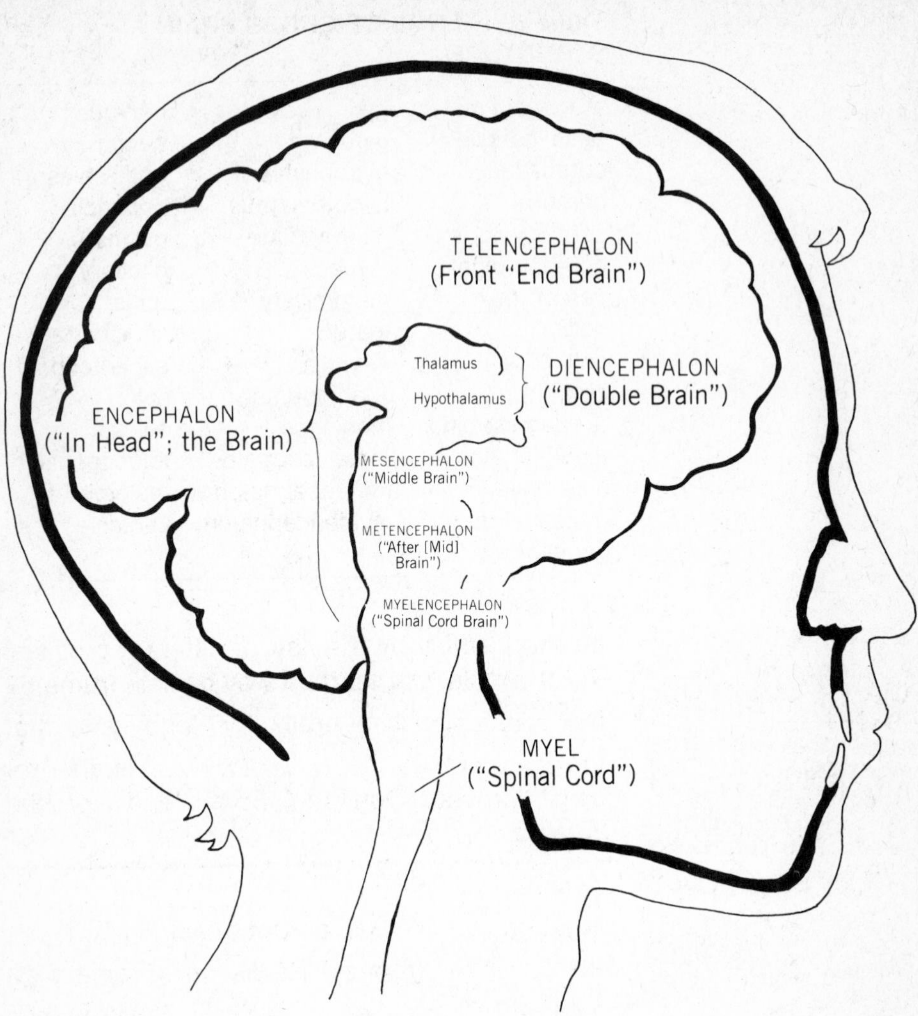

Figure 6.1. MAIN BRAIN DIVISIONS

brain cerebr/um (ser′ ə brəm, sə rē′ brəm)	**626** *Cerebr*, like *encephal*, means "__________." While *encephal* takes *-on*, this root uses the ending of *capitulum* (frame 513) as its "presence of" suffix. Consequently, __________/____, like *encephal/on*, means "presence of the brain."
cerebrum	**627** The ______________ is the main mass of

"brain" tissue "present within the head." Hence its identical meaning to *encephalon*.

628

telencephalon

The cerebrum develops from the immature ______________ (front "end brain," frame 624).

629

cerebr/al (ser′ ə brəl, sə rē′ brəl)

Cerebr combines with the "referring to" suffix of *neural* (frame 621) to make ________/____ ("referring to the main brain mass").

630

cerebral

The ______________ ("main brain mass") surface is covered by an external layer of nervous tissue.

631

cerebral cortex

cerebrum

Cortex (kôr′ teks) comes directly from the entire Latin term for "bark" or "rind." Like the rough "bark" on a tree or the pitted "rind" covering the soft inner meat of an orange, the ______________* forms a thin irregular surface mantle for the delicate ______________ ("main brain mass").

632

-us

Have you ever closely examined the bark on an old gnarled tree trunk? Visualize it with your cerebrum. You see a wavy pattern of raised ridges and deep furrows. These concepts are represented by the following roots:

gyr "circle" or "ring"
sulc "furrow, ditch, or wrinkle"

Both of these roots take ______, the "presence of" suffix found within *rectus* (frame 600).

633

Gyr/us (jī′ rəs)

sulc/us (sul′ kəs)

______/____ means "presence of a circle or ring," while ________/____ means "presence of a furrow, ditch, or wrinkle."

---

gyrus sulcus	**634** Each __________ (sulcus/gyrus) is a raised ridge "present" on the cerebrum that partially "encircles" the surface of the main brain mass in a broken interrupted "ring." Each __________ (sulcus/gyrus) is a deep "furrow" or valley "present" between these raised mountainous crescents of cerebral cortex.
gyri (jī′ rī) sulci (sul′ sī)	**635** Terms ending in *-us* form plurals with -i. Thus __________ are raised semicircular folds of cerebrum, while __________ are the steep ditches between them.
mening/es (me nin′ jēz)	**636** *Mening* is a root for "membrane," and it takes the suffix found in *oblique* (frame 600). The __________/____ are "membranes present" over both the cerebral cortex and the rest of the central nervous system.
meninges	**637** Like a protective mother or mater (term for "mother" in Latin) these __________ ("membranes") form a secure wrapping for the fragile neural tissue.
maters (mā′ tərz) -oid	**638** The meninges seem to have the personalities of different types of human __________ ("mothers"). Pia (pē′ ə) is a Latin term for "gentle." Conversely *dura* (dyoor′ ə) is the term for "hard" or "tough." And *arachn* (ə rak′ n-) is a root for "spider's web." Recall that __________ is a suffix meaning "resembling," as in "resembling a socket" (frame 475).
dura mater meninge	**639** The __________* ("tough mother") is a whitish leathery fibrous __________

("membrane") that forms the *durable* external covering for the central nervous system.

---

arachnoid (ə rak′ noid) mater	**640** The ______________________* ("spider mother") is the middle membrane, which has delicate fibers "resembling a spider's web."
pia mater	**641** The ______________* ("gentle mother") is the delicate inner membrane that clings *tenderly* to the nervous tissue itself (Fig. 6.2).

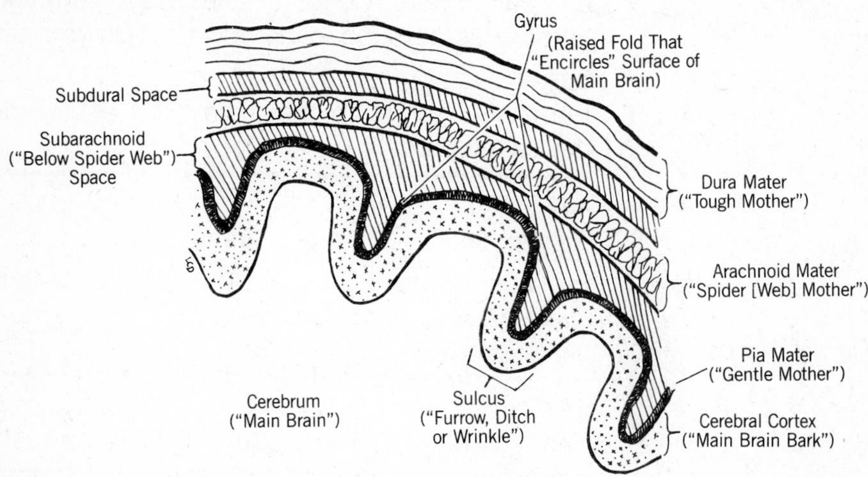

Figure 6.2. MENINGES ("MEMBRANES") COVERING THE CENTRAL NERVOUS SYSTEM

Sub- sub/arachn/oid (sub′ ə rak′ noid)	**642** ________, the prefix in *subcutaneous* (frame 394) means "beneath." Consequently ______/ ____________/______ translates as "beneath the spider-web resembler."
subarachnoid pia mater	**643** The ________________ *space* is the hollow area "beneath the arachnoid" membrane but above the ____________* ("tender mother") (Fig. 6.2).

spinal cord	**644** *Spin* like *myel* (frame 625) is a root for "________________."* It often combines with the suffix of *intercostal* (frame 585) to make adjectival terms.
Spin/al	**645** ________/____ means "referring to the spinal cord."
Cerebr cerebr/o/spin/al (ser′ e brō spī′ nəl)	**646** __________, the root indicating the idea of a "main brain mass" (frame 629), generally takes o as its connecting vowel. Thus you can build __________/__/________/____, a term that "refers to the main brain mass and the spinal cord."
ventr ventric/le (ven′ tri kəl)	**647** *Ventric* like __________ (frame 102) is a root for "belly." Thus ____________/____ means "little belly" just as *fascicle* (frame 531) means "little bundle."
ventricles subarachnoid cerebrospinal	**648** The ________________ ("little bellies") are hollow chambers in and around the central nervous system. Both these chambers and the ________________ space between the arachnoid mater and the pia mater are filled with circulating ________________ ______ ("brain-spinal cord") fluid.
telencephalon	**649** In addition to the cerebrum and a number of ventricles containing nourishing and protective cerebrospinal fluid, the ______________ ________ ("end brain," frame 624) also includes the *basal ganglia* (gang′ glē ə).
Bas/al	**650** ______/_____ probably means "referring to the bottom or base." And since *mitochondria*

gangli/on; -on (gang′ glē on or gang′ glē ən)	(frame 246) is the plural of *mitochondrion*, it only stands to reason that *ganglia* is the plural of ____________/____. The suffix _____ is the "presence of" ending that occurs in the singular form of both *mitochondria* and *ganglia*.
basal ganglia	**651** *Gangli* is a Greek root for "knot." Therefore the __________________________* are small masses or tight "knots" of closely packed nerve cells "present" near the "base" of the cerebrum.
diencephalon hypothalam	**652** So far we have been mainly discussing the parts of the telencephalon. Recall from frame 625 that the ________________________ is the "double-brain," consisting as it does of "two" major "brain" areas. These are partially described as *thalam* "bedroom" or "inner chamber" and the ____________________ "below the bedroom or inner chamber." (Use the prefix found in *hypodermis*, not the one in *subdermis*, frame 393.)
-us	**653** Both of the partial terms in frame 652 are made complete by the addition of _____, the suffix also occurring within *trapezius* (frame 579).
thalam/us (thal′ ə məs) hypo/thalam/us (hī′ pō thal′ ə məs)	**654** Thus the ____________/____ is a "bedroom or inner chamber present" in the brain, while the ________/____________/____ is the brain region "present" immediately "below" this "bedroom" (Fig. 6.3).
middle midsagittal	**655** *Mid-* like *medi-* and *mes-* (frames 152–153) means "____________." And the __________ ____________ plane (frame 152) exactly di-

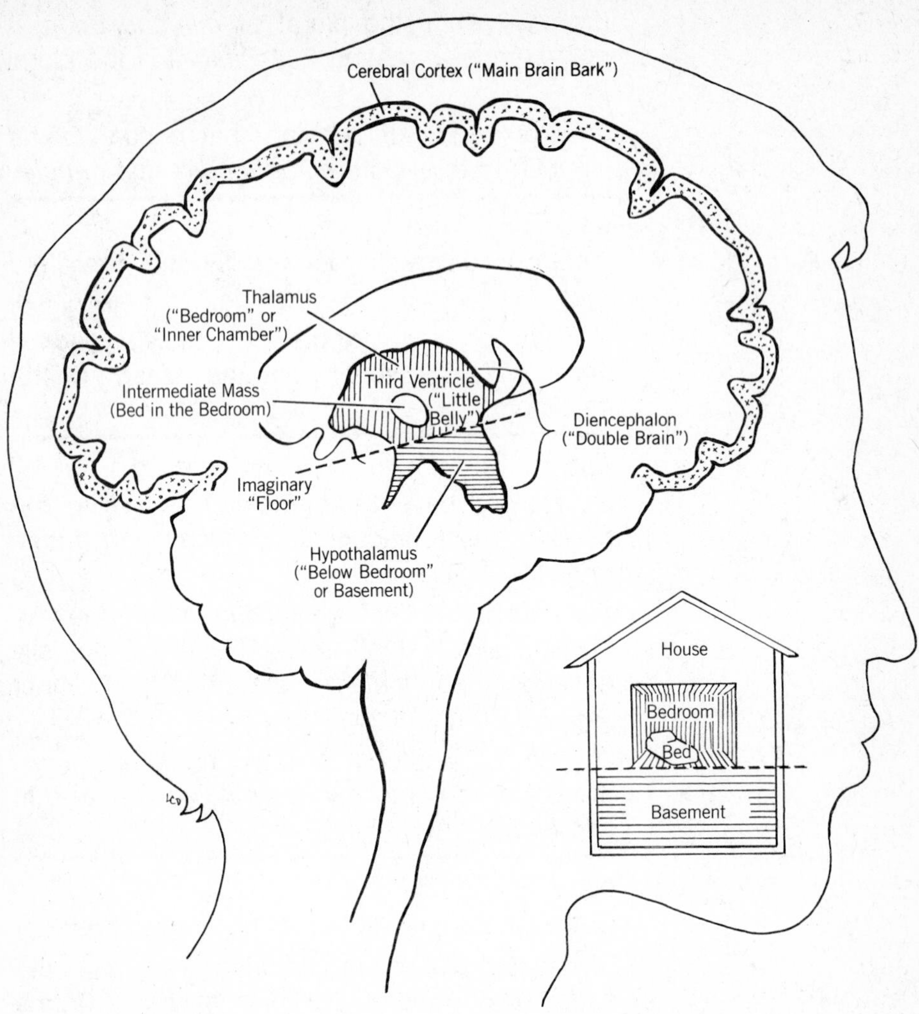

Figure 6.3. MIDSAGITTAL SECTION THROUGH BRAIN

section diencephalon	vides the body into right and left pieces of equal size. When an actual ____________ ("process of cutting," frame 133) is made through this plane, the interior of the ________________ ("double brain" = thalamus + hypothalamus) can be seen (Fig. 6.3).
thalamus	**656** Examination of Figure 6.3 does indeed reveal that the ____________ is like a bedroom

hypothalamus	or inner chamber deep within the brain. If the *brain* is a *house*, and the *thalamus* is a *bedroom* on the ground floor, then the ________ ________________ must be the *basement*!
ventricle	**657** Both the thalamus and hypothalamus are like rooms in that they include a hollow area called the *third* ________________ ("little belly," frame 647).
bed intermediate mass	**658** By definition if the thalamus is a *bedroom* it must contain a ______! Figure 6.3 shows a small oval *bed*-shaped "mass" located in an "intermediate" position within the thalamus. Not surprisingly, this centrally located structure is called the ________________________ ________,* named literally according to its "middle" position "between" the roof of the thalamus above and the floor of the hypothalamus below it.
thalamus	**659** The *intermediate mass* is considered part of the ________________ (thalamus/hypothalamus).
hypothalamus	**660** But the ________________________ ("presence below the bedroom") has a number of notable structures clearly visible on its ventral surface (Fig. 6.4).
	661 Facts for properly naming these structures are given below: *chiasm* term for Greek letter "X" or "chi" *optic* complete term for "eye" *hypophys* root meaning "undergrowth" *pituit* root for "mucus" or "phlegm"

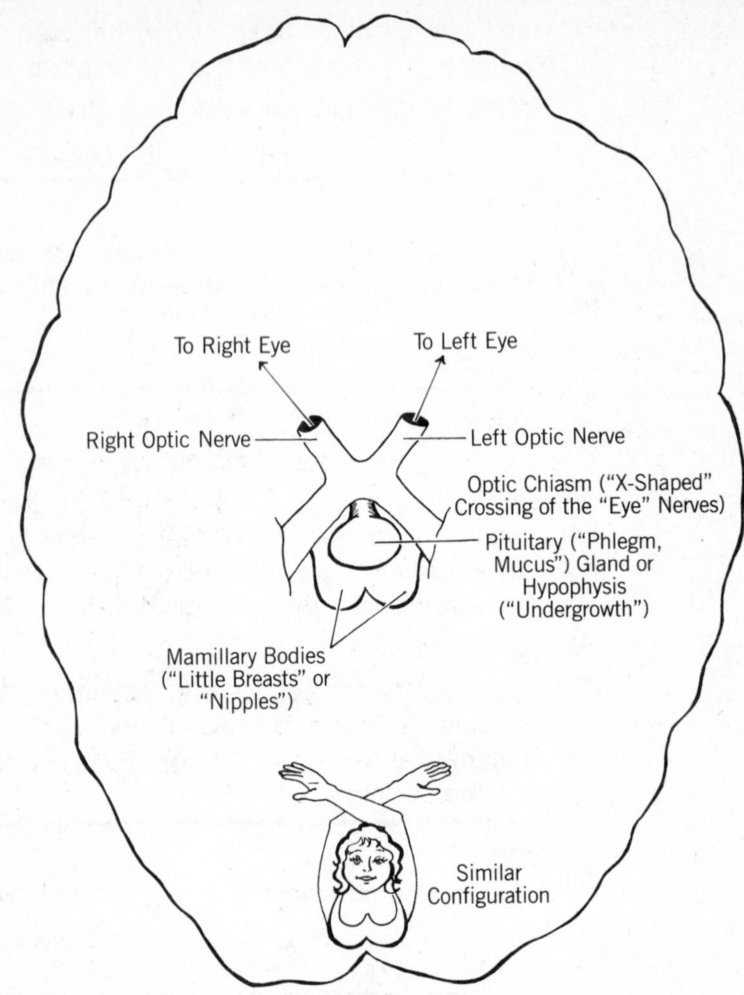

Figure 6.4. FLOOR OF THE HYPOTHALAMUS— VENTRAL VIEW OF CEREBRUM

mammill root indicating "little breasts," that is, "nipples"

-ary	In frame 444 you learned that ______, the suffix in *medullary*, means "pertaining to." However it also means "characterized by" in other cases.
-is	And recall that ______, the suffix in *femoris* (frame 584), means "presence of."

662

Now employ the information of the preceding

hypophys/is
(hī pof′ i sis)
pituit/ary
(pi tyo͞o′ i ter ē)
mammill/ary
(mam′ i ler ē)
optic chiasm
(op′ tik kī′ az əm)

learning frame to test your skills in word-building: ________/____ "presence of an undergrowth," ________/_____ "characterized by mucus/phlegm," ________/_____ "characterized by nipples," ______________* "X or chi" associated with the "eye."

---

optic chiasm

663
Actually the ________________* is simply the "X"-shaped or "chi"-shaped union of the *optic nerves* carrying sensory impulses from both "eyes" (Fig. 6.4).

---

pituitary

664
The ______________ *gland*, according to ancient belief, was "characterized by mucus or phlegm." This name apparently derived from the notion that the thick slimy mucus of the nose was actually channeled there from this particular gland, which reportedly secreted it.

---

hypophysis

665
This false impression was really not as unreasonable as we with twentieth century hindsight might at first suppose. The pituitary gland was also called the ______________, or "undergrowth present" on the floor of the main brain mass. *Galen* (gā′ lən), the famous Greek physician and "Father of Experimental Physiology," wrote about this pituitary or brain "undergrowth" less than 200 years after the death of Christ!

---

hypophysis

666
It apparently seemed logical to ancient thinkers that the ______________, which appeared to "grow" out from "under" the base

of the hypothalamus and which was attached to it by a narrow stalk, might also secrete mucus into the nostrils.

pituitary sella turcica sphenoid	**667** Indeed, the ______ ("characterized by mucus") *gland* does lie hidden within the ______* ("Turkish saddle," frame 494) of the ______ ("wedgelike," frame 475) bone, not too far behind the nose!
mammillary	**668** Finally, the ______ *bodies*, two small rounded structures bulging out with the "characteristics" of "little breasts," protrude like a pair of tiny "nipples" from the soft underbelly of the hypothalamus (Fig. 6.4).
mesencephalon encephalons	**669** Certainly no one can accuse the early anatomists of having dull imaginations! Less vivid mental gymnastics are required to name the ______ ("middle brain," frame 625). This region is called the *mid*brain because it stands below two different ______ ("within heads" or "brains," frame 623) and above two others (Fig. 6.1).
collicul/us (kol ik′ yə ləs) -us	**670** The dorsal aspect of the midbrain sports a set of four little hills. *Collicul* means "little hill" and consequently ______/____ translates as "presence of a little hill," where the suffix is that used in *sulcus* (frame 633). Remember that singular terms ending with ______ form plurals using *-i*.
collicul/i (kol ik′ yə lī)	**671** Consequently, ______/__ are "little hills" just as *sulc/i* (frame 635) are "wrinkles."

superior colliculi

inferior colliculi

672
Figure 6.5 reveals that there are two larger upper ______________________* (superior colliculi/medial colliculi/inferior colliculi) and two smaller lower ______________________* (superior colliculli/medial colliculi/inferior colliculi) present on the midbrain like four humps on the back of a camel (Fig. 6.5).

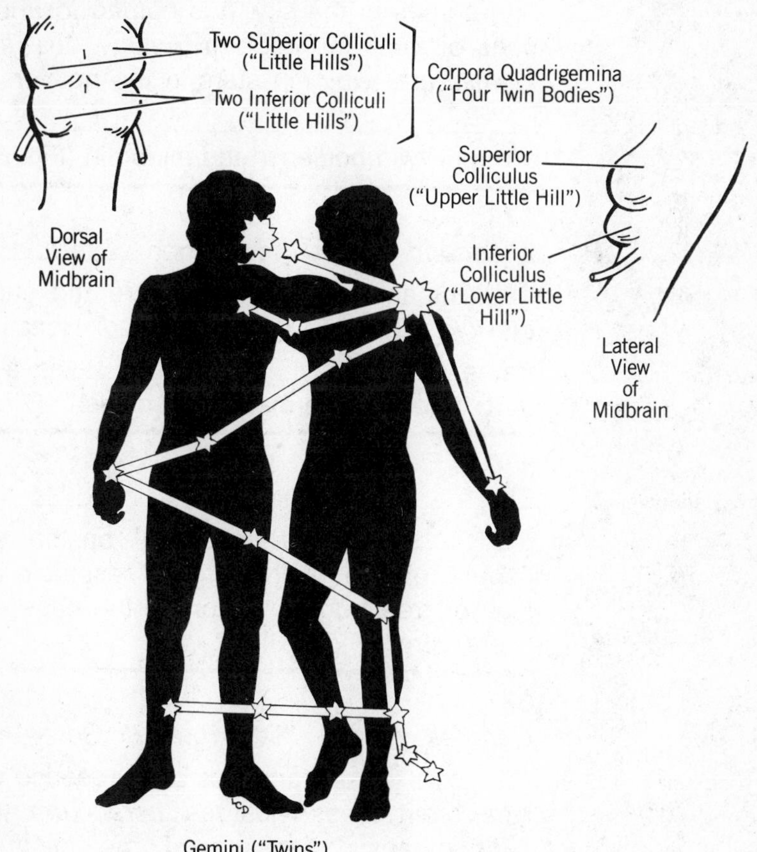

Figure 6.5. THE STORY OF **GEMINI**

quadri-

673
Corpor/a (kôr′ pər ə) are "bodies" and *gemin/a* (jem′ i nə) are "twins." Recall that ____________, the prefix in *quadriceps* (frame 596),

quadrigemina (kwäd ri jem′ i nə) | means "four." Thus ____________ means "four twins." And the two superior colliculi "twins" plus the two inferior colliculi

corpora quadrigemina | "twins" make up the ____________ ____________* ("four twin bodies") of the mesencephalon (Fig. 6.5).

674

The *Gemini* "twins" is the third sign of the zodiac and a constellation featuring a pair of bright stars in the sky. It is named for the twin sons of Zeus in Greek mythology. Just as the *Gemini* are two twin stars in the heavens, the ____________* are four twin bodies in the midbrain (Fig. 6.5).

corpora quadrigemina

675

peduncle/le (ped′ əng kəl) | If *pedunc* means "foot" then ____________/ ____ means "little foot," where the suffix in *clavicle* (frame 611) is employed. Recall from

cerebral | frame 629 that ____________ is a term that "refers to the main brain mass."

676

cerebral peduncles | The ____________ ____________* are two "little feet" on the ventral aspect of the midbrain that resemble small legs or tree trunks supporting the base of the "cerebrum" (Fig. 6.6).

677

cerebell/um (ser ə bel′ əm) | *Cerebell* means "little brain." So ____________ ____________/____ translates as "presence of the little brain mass" just as *cerebr/um* (frame 626) means "presence of the main brain mass."

678

cerebellum | The ____________ is the "little brain mass present" on the dorsal aspect of the brainstem. It is attached to the stem by a num-

peduncles | ber of ____________ ("little feet"). A

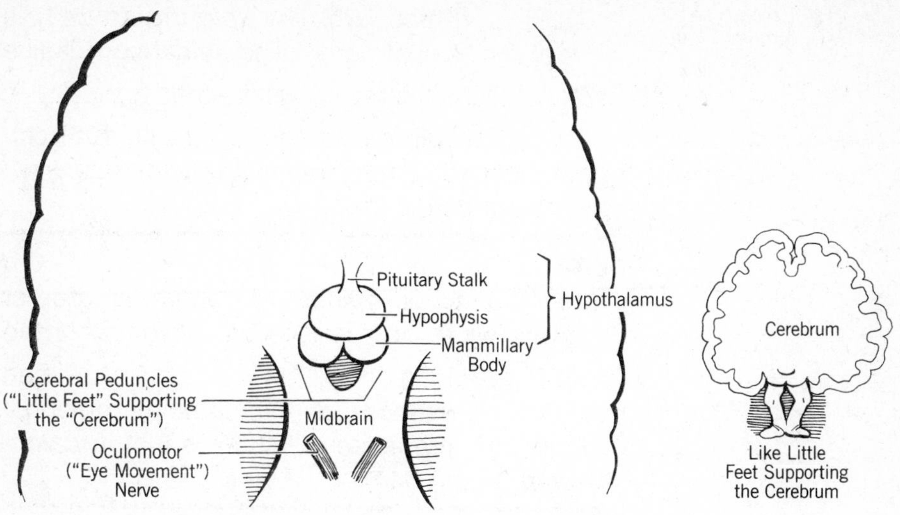

Figure 6.6. PEDUNCLES ("LITTLE FEET")

metencephalon gyri sulci	derivative of the ______________ ("after brain," frame 625), it does somewhat resemble the cerebrum in that it has both ________ ("circular" folds, frame 635) and __________ ("furrows") on its surface.
midbrain transverse	**679** *Pons* (ponz, pons) means "bridge." This structure appears as a big bulge on the ventral aspect of the lower brainstem, inferior to the ______________ (mesencephalon). It contains many ______________ (frames 131–132) or horizontal fibers that "turn across" the midline like a nervous "bridge."
cerebellum pons metencephalon	**680** Both the ______________ ("little cerebrum") and the ________ ("bridge" of transverse fibers) originate from the ______________ ("after brain").
medull	**681** Recall that ____________ (frame 445) is a root representing "middle" and "marrow." And

myel

vertebral

_______ (frame 625) like *spin* (frame 644) is a root for "spinal cord." The spinal cord is like soft whitish "marrow" within the _______ _______ ("jointed backbone," frame 106) column, consequently *medull*=*myel*="marrow" or "spinal cord."

Oblongat/a (ob long gä′ tə)

682
If something is *oblong* its length is greater than its width or it is tapered. *Oblongat* is the root for "oblong." _______/__ then means "presence of (something) oblong," where the "presence of" suffix is that in *sarcolemma* (frame 544).

Medull/a (mə dul′ ə)

683
_______/__ likewise translates as "presence of a middle, marrow, or spinal cord."

---

medulla oblongata

684
Putting the new information of the last two frames together, construct two terms that indicate "presence of something oblong" leading into the "spinal cord": _______ _______.*

---

medulla oblongata

myelencephalon

685
The _______* represents the "tapered oblong" upward continuation of the "spinal cord" into the base of the skull. It derives from the _______ _______ ("spinal cord brain," frame 625) and thus logically is involved as a center for many vital *spinal* reflexes.

---

cerebrum

686
In summation, the human brain is like one gigantic mushroom. The wrinkled spongy *cap* of the mushroom is represented by the _______ _______ ("major brain tissue mass"). And like the *stem* of a mushroom, which plugs into the bottom of the *cap*, the top of the *brainstem*,

thalamus medulla oblongata	represented by the ________ ("bedroom," frame 654), fits into the bottom of the *cerebrum*. The brain is a mushroom whose stem narrows at its tapered base, the ________ ________.*

Table 6.2 SELECTED TERMINOLOGY OF NERVES, TRACTS, AND MICROSCOPIC NEUROANATOMY

abducent	hypoglossal	Ranvier
acoustic	internode	sensory
afferent	motor	somatic
auditory	myelin	spinocerebellar
autonomic	neurilemma	spinothalamic
axon	neurium	sympathetic
corticospinal	neuroglia	synapse
dendrite	neuron	synaptic vesicles
efferent	nodes	trigeminal
endoneurium	oculomotor	trochlear
epineurium	olfactory	vagus
femoral	parasympa-thetic	vestibulo-cochlear
glossopha-ryngeal	perineurium	

encephalon vertebral	**687** If the ________ ("presence within the head," frame 623) resembles a mushroom, then the spinal cord is like a long narrow root with many branches or "spines" firmly anchoring the mushroom in the "ground" of the ________ ("referring to jointed backbone," frame 106) canal.
neur neur/on (nyo͞o′ ron) -on	**688** Each of these branches entering or leaving the spinal cord is a *nerve*. Recall from frame 621 that ________, like *nerv*, is a root for "nerve." Consequently, ________/____ indicates "presence of a nerve," where ______, the suffix within *encephalon* (frame 52), is used.
	689 Nerves derive from the fiberlike processes of

many individual nerve cells, hence the term ______________ ("presence of nerve") for these cells.

neuron

690

Just as a skeletal muscle consists of ______________ ("little bundles," frame 531) of individual *muscle* fibers, a body nerve consists of ______________ ("little bundles") of individual ______________ (muscle/nerve/connective tissue) fibers (Fig. 6.7).

fascicles

fascicles

nerve

691

And just as ____/__/____ (frame 526) denotes "presence of a muscle," ______/__/____ denotes "presence of a nerve." As you can see, many of the terms involving muscle also apply to nerves!

mys/i/um

neur/i/um (nyo͞o′ rē əm)

692

For example, ______________ is the layer of fascia that is "present upon" the outer surface of a "nerve," just as ______________ (frame 528) is the layer of fascia "present upon" the outer surface of a "muscle" (Figs. 5.1 and 6.7).

epineurium (ep i nyo͞o′ rē əm)

epimysium

693

And ______________ is the layer of fascia that is "present around" individual fascicles of "nerve" fibers, in the same manner that ______________ (frame 529) is the fascia "present around" individual fascicles of "muscle" fibers. (Contrast Figs. 6.7 and 5.1.)

perineurium (per i nyo͞o′ rē əm)

perimysium

694

Finally, ______________ is the fascia "present within" the bundles of little "nerve" fibers, in the identical way that ______________ (frame 530) is the fascia "pres-

endoneurium (en dō nyo͞o′ rē əm)

endomysium

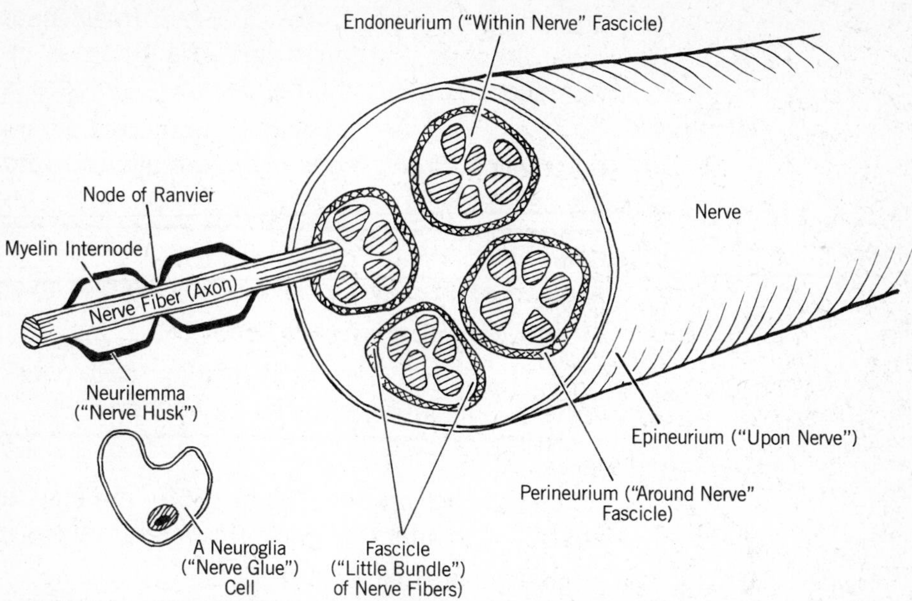

Figure 6.7. CROSS-SECTION OF A NERVE

ent within" little bundles of "muscle" fibers. (Compare Fig. 6.7 with Fig. 5.1.)

---

i
neur/i/lemm/a
(nyo͞o ri lem' ə)
sarc/o/lemm/a

695
In the last few frames *neur* has used the combining vowel __; so too when we discuss the ________/__/________/__ ("nerve husk presence") as the counterpart to the ________/__/________/__ ("flesh husk presence," frame 544) (Figs. 5.2 and 6.7).

---

ax
Dendrit/e (den' drīt)
-e
Ax/on (aks' on)

696
Dendrit means "tree" and ____ (frame 410) is the root for "axle or axis." ____________/__ means "presence of a tree," where ____, the "presence of" suffix in *meninge* (frame 636), is borrowed. ____/____ means "presence of an axis," where the suffix of *neuron* is borrowed.

697
Each neuron generally has several processes

axon dendrites	branching off from it. An ________ (main neuronal process that forms an "axis") carries information away from the cell body, whereas ________________ (highly branched fibers resembling "trees") convey information toward the cell body.
neurilemma	**698** A given axon may be covered by both a layer of *myelin* (mī′ ə lin) and one of __________ __________ ("nerve husk") (Fig. 6.7). Conversely, it might be covered by neither!
marrow	**699** The suffix in *myosin* (frame 559) means "a neutral substance." And *myel* (frame 681) means either "spinal cord" or "____________."
Myel/in lipid	**700** ________/____ ("neutral substance in marrow") is a white __________ ("fatty," frame 303) material. Like the yellow "marrow" deep within long bones, this substance is primarily fatty in nature. Hence the same root for both.
neur/o/gli/a (nyo͞o rog′ lē ə)	**701** *Gli* is Greek for "glue." Using the root in *neuron* plus the connecting vowel "o," build a term for "presence of nerve glue": ________/ __/______/__. Employ the suffix located in *neurilemma* (frame 695).
neuroglia myelin	**702** The __________________ are a group of various types of connective tissue cells "present" in the "nervous" system that in a sense "glue" the parts of the system together. Certain types of these cells also produce ____________ ("a neutral substance in marrow").
	703 A *node* is a "gap" between adjacent beads of myelin on an axon. These gaps are called

Answers	Frames
Ranvier (rän vē ā′)	*nodes of* ______, after their French discoverer, Louis Ranvier.
inter- internode	**704** Remember that ______, the prefix in *intermediate* (frame 658), means "between." Thus ______ means "between a gap."
internodes	**705** The myelin ______ are the beads "between" the "gaps" called *nodes of Ranvier* (Fig. 6.7).
axon ions nodes	**706** Nervous impulses are conducted down the ______ (dendrite/axon) *away from* the neuron cell body. Na^+ and Cl^- ______ (atoms/ions/molecules) and other charged particles "go" through the neuron membrane at the ______ (nodes/internodes) of Ranvier, "carrying" (frame 262) an electric current.
synaps/e (sin′ aps)	**707** *Synaps* means "coming together," so ______/__ is the "presence of a coming together," where *-e* is the appropriate suffix.
synapse	**708** The ______ is the place where neurons "come together." But this place of union is actually just a narrow fluid-filled space, because the neurons in the human make no direct physical contact.
vesicles	**709** The neuron, like many other cells, contains ______ ("little bladders," frame 240).
-ic	**710** *Synapt,* like *synaps*, is a "coming together." And ______, the suffix in *optic* (frame 663), means "pertaining to." Consequently, ______

synaptic vesicles	______________________* are "little bladders" that "refer to" the place where neurons "come together."
synaptic vesicles synapse axon	**711** These ______________________ ______* are "tiny bladder"-like sacs containing a special chemical transmitter substance that is released into the ____________ (site of neuron union) after an electrical message is conducted to the terminal end of the ________ ("presence of an axle," frame 696).
ad- af-	**712** *Affer* derives from the prefix ______, "toward" as in *adductor* (frame 571), plus the root *fer*, "to carry." In this case ______ is equivalent to *ad-*.
-ent af/fer/ent (af′ ər ənt)	**713** Recall that ________, the suffix in *nutrient* (frame 516), means "one that." Thus ____/ ______/______ means "one that carries toward."
ex- ef/fer/ent (ef′ ər ənt)	**714** *Ef-*, like the prefix ______ (Table 4, frame 42), means "out of" or "away from." Consequently, ____/______/______ means "one that carries away from."
Afferent efferent	**715** ______________ (Afferent/Efferent) nerves are those that "carry" sensory impulses "toward" the central nervous system. And ____ __________ (afferent/efferent) nerves "carry" motor messages "away from" the brain and spinal cord.
	716 Efferent nerves pass from the central nervous system out to the heart, stomach, and other

viscera	______________ ("internal organs," frame 85). These "motor" nerves cause contractions or secretions in the internal organs they stimulate, as if they were really a *motor*!
auto/nom/ic (ô tə nom′ ik)	**717** *Auto* is a prefix for "self," while *nom* is a root for "regulating" that takes the suffix of *synaptic* (frame 710). The activity of the motor nerves supplying the viscera can be described as ________/________/____ ("self-regulating") in nature.
sympathetic	**718** If you have *sympathy* for a person you are literally ______________________ to his/her plight. These two highlighted terms come directly from the Greek for "suffering with."
para- parasympathetic sympathetic	**719** According to Table 4 (frame 42) __________, like *par-*, is a prefix for "beside." Thus the ______________________________ nerves are those which lie "beside" the __________ ____________ ("suffering with") nerves.
sympathetic parasympathetic autonomic	**720** Both the ______________________ ("suffering with") nerves and the ____________ ______________ ("beside suffering with") nerves belong to the ________________ portion of the nervous system, since their activity is largely beyond our voluntary control.
motor parasympathetic	**721** The sympathetic nerves are efferent or __________ (sensory/motor) nerves that run to practically all of the viscera, with the ______________________________ nerves running right along "beside" them.

sympathetic

722
The ______________ (sympathetic/parasympathetic) nerves are generally most active when a person is "suffering with" stress or arousal.

somat/ic (sō mat' ik)

723
If *somat* is a root for "body" then ________/____ means "pertaining to the body," where the suffix in *sympathetic* is employed.

somatic

724
The ______________ ("body") portion of the nervous system consists of both afferent and efferent nerves supplying the skin and skeletal muscles, which make up the main *body* "wall."

somatic

725
The ______________ (autonomic/somatic) system is considered "voluntary" in nature, since stimulation of skeletal muscles is often done with our conscious control.

somatic

726
Individual peripheral nerves in the ______________ (autonomic/somatic) nervous system are generally named for the areas of skin and skeletal muscle they supply.

femor/al (fem' ər əl)

727
For example, the __________/____ ("pertaining to thigh;" use root in frame 583 plus *-al*) nerve supplies the skin and skeletal muscles of the anterior portion of the *thigh*.

cranial

trochle

728
The ______________ ("skull," frame 32) nerves are likewise named for their locations, functions, or resemblances. Below is a list of some of the roots found in the names of these nerves:

__________ "pulley" (frame 509)
gloss "tongue"
ocul "eye"

audit "hear"
acoust "hear"
vag "wander"
olfact "smell"
pharynge "throat"
cochle "snail shell"
vestibul "little entrance room"

729

Observe and pronounce this partial list of cranial nerves:

glossopharyngeal (glos′ō fa rin′ jē əl)
hypoglossal (hī pō glos′ əl)
vestibulocochlear (ves tib′ yə lo kok′ lē ər)
auditory (ô′ di tôr ē)
acoustic (ə ko͞o′ tik)
abducent (ab dyo͞o′ sənt)
olfactory (ōl fak′ tər ē)
vagus (vā′ gəs)
trigeminal (trī jem′ i nəl)
trochlear (trok′ lē ər)

730

Now try to match the names of these cranial nerves with their literal translations below:

vestibul/o/cochle/ar
vag/us
hypo/gloss/al
gloss/o/pharynge/al
acoust/ic
audit/ory
tri/gemin/al
olfact/ory
ab/duc/ent
trochle/ar

__________/___/__________/____ "pertains to a little entrance room and a snail shell (in the ear)," ______/____ "presence of a wanderer," ________/__________/_____ "refers to (something) under the tongue," __________/___/______________/_____ "pertains to the tongue and throat," __________/____ "pertains to hearing," ________/______ "characterized by hearing," ____/________/____ "refers to three twin (nerve roots)," __________/______ "characterized by smelling," _____/_______/______ "one that moves (the eyeball) away from (the body midline)" (see frame 571), ____________/____ "refers to a pulley (ac-

ocul/o/motor

tion on the eyeball)," ______/___/___ ___ the main "eyeball mover."

-ory

731
Note that both *auditory* and *olfactory* end with ______, a suffix that, like *-ary*, means "characterized by."

---

acoustic

auditory

732
And the three names of ________, ________, and *vestibulocochlear* all represent the same eighth cranial nerve, the nerve of hearing. (Glance ahead at Fig. 7.2, if desired.)

---

vagus

parasympathetic

733
The ______ or 10th cranial nerve is the major branch of the ________ ________ system that "wanders beside the suffering with" nerves to supply many of the viscera.

---

sens/ory

734
Tracts of ascending and descending nerve fibers staying within the central nervous system are commonly named according to their places of origin and destination. For example, both the *spinocerebellar* (spī′ nō ser ə bel′ ər) and the *spinothalamic* (spī′ nō thə lam′ ik) *tracts* contain ascending _____/_____ ("characterized by *sens*ation") nerve fibers rather than descending motor fibers.

---

spin/o/thalam/ic

735
The _____/__/______/___ tract is the one that carries sensory messages from the *spinal* cord up to the "bedroom" (frame 654) of the brain.

---

spin/o/cerebell/ar

736
And the _____/__/________/ ___ tract is the one conducting sensory mes-

sages from the *spinal* cord up to the "little brain mass" (frame 677).

737

cerebrospinal	Recall that *cerebr/o* represents the "cerebrum" and that it is ______ ______ ("pertaining to the cerebrum and spinal cord," frame 646) fluid that circulates through the ventricles.

738

cortic/o/spin/al (kôr′ ti kō spī′ nəl)	In a similar manner, *cortic/o* represents the "cortex" of the cerebrum and ______/__/______/____ is a term that "refers to the cortex and the spinal cord."

739

corticospinal	The ______ tract arises from motor areas of the cerebral *cortex* and descends to the level of the *spinal* cord.

Now do the Self-Test for Unit 6 (page 273 in the Appendix).

UNIT 7
TERMS OF THE EYE AND EAR

pinn/a (pin′ ə) corne	**740** *Pinn* means "wing," and ________/__ is a term for "presence of a wing," where the suffix is the same as that in *medulla* (frame 684). Here are some other roots that take this particular "presence of" ending: *palpebr* "winker" *retin* "net" *fove* "pit" *conjunctiv* "bind together" __________ "horny" (frame 399) *scler* "hard" *lute* "yellow" *macul* "spot"
pinna	**741** The __________ is the external "wing present" on the side of the head. This outer portion of the ear is like a deep dish for catching and amplifying sound waves.
palpebra (pal′ pə brə)	**742** The ______________ or *eyelid* is the external "winker present" over the soft sphere of the eyeball.
conjunctiva (kon jungk tī′ və) palpebra	**743** The ______________________ is a mucous membrane "present" as a thin film over the anterior surface of the eyeball and as an inner lining for the ________________ (eyelid). It acts to "bind" eyeball and eyelid "together."

Table 7.1 BASIC TERMS OF THE EYE AND EAR

aqueous	incus	pupil
aqueous humor	iris	retina
auricle	labyrinth	saccule
choroid	macula lutea	sclera
ciliary	malleus	stapes
cochlea	meatus	tympanic
conjunctiva	organ of Corti	utricle
cornea	ossicle	vitreous
fovea centralis	palpebra	vitreous humor
humor	pinna	

744

conjunctiva

cornea (kôr′ nē ə)

sclera (sklir′ ə, skler′ ə)

The ______________ ("binder") covers the thicker transparent ______________ "present" as a "horny coat" over the anterior aspect of the eye. Posteriorly, this coat is "present" as the "hard" tough ______________ or *white of the eye* (Fig. 7.1).

745

retina (ret′ ən ə)

synapses

Internal to all the aforementioned structures, deep in the back of the eye, there is the ______________, the innermost layer of the eyeball wall "present" as a delicate "net" of visual receptor cells. These cells, some shaped like *rods* and *cones*, form a complex "net" by "coming together" at places of union called ______________ (frame 707).

746

macula lutea (mak′ yoo lə lyōō′ tē ə or lōō′ tē ə)

retina

You should surmise from frame 740 that the ______________* is a "yellowish spot present" on the ______________ ("net") (Fig. 7.1).

747

Central/is

______________/______ means "presence of (something) central," just as *abdominis* (frame 584) means "presence of the abdomen." Glancing back at frame 740 one last time, you

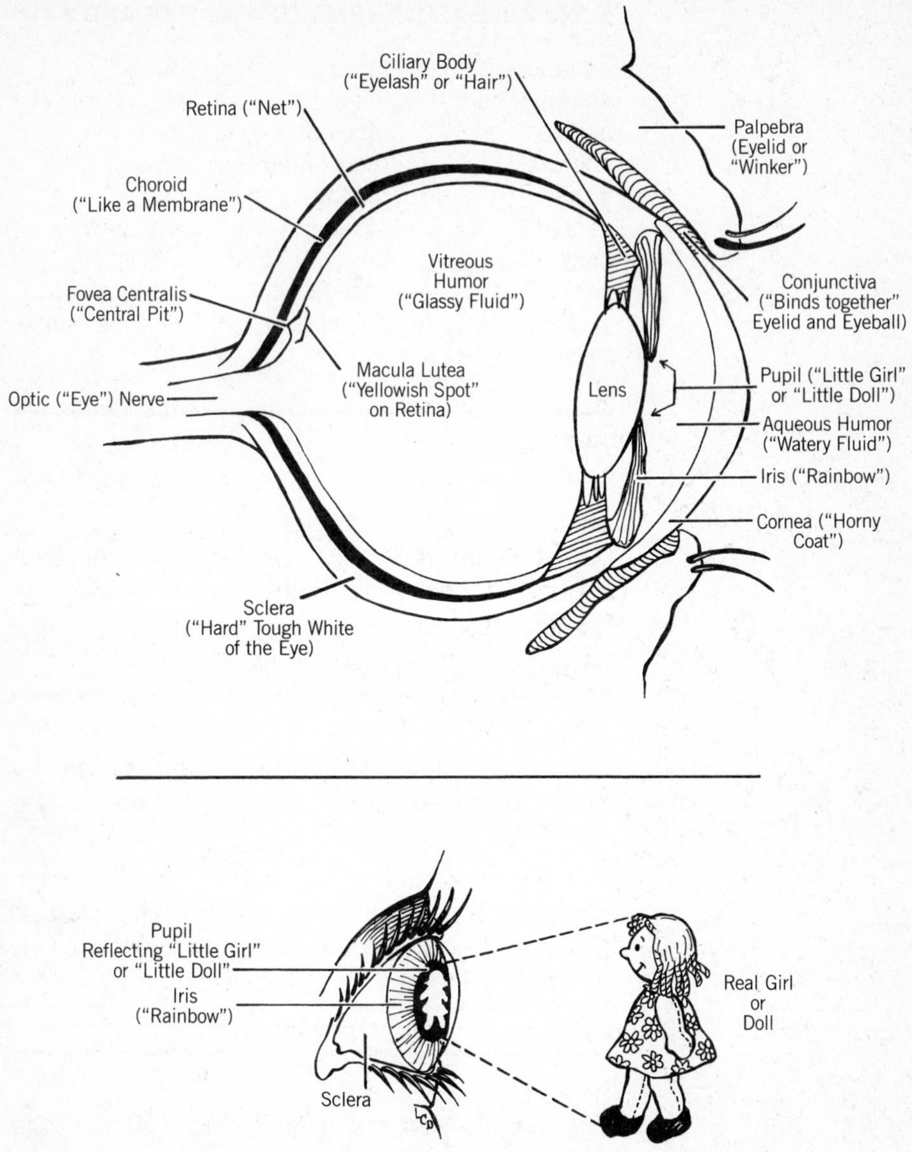

Ciliary Body
("Eyelash" or "Hair")
Retina ("Net")
Palpebra
(Eyelid or
"Winker")
Choroid
("Like a Membrane")
Vitreous
Humor
("Glassy Fluid")
Fovea Centralis
("Central Pit")
Conjunctiva
("Binds together"
Eyelid and Eyeball)
Macula Lutea
("Yellowish Spot"
on Retina)
Lens
Pupil ("Little Girl"
or "Little Doll")
Optic ("Eye") Nerve
Aqueous Humor
("Watery Fluid")
Iris ("Rainbow")
Cornea ("Horny
Coat")
Sclera
("Hard" Tough White
of the Eye)

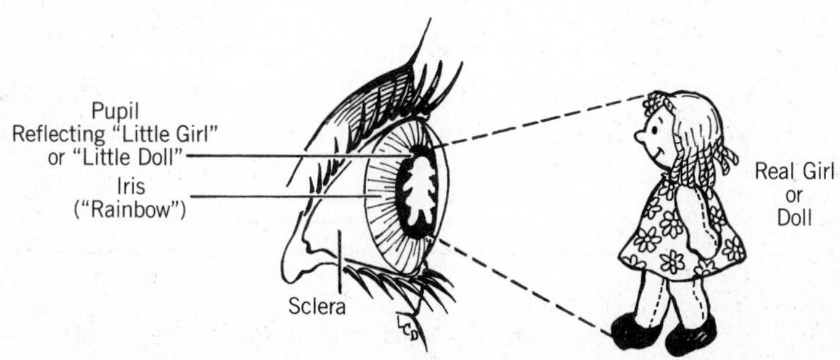

Figure 7.1. LATERAL VIEW OF EYEBALL INTERIOR

fovea (fō′ vē ə) centralis	should deduce that ______________* translates as "presence of a central pit."
fovea centralis	**748** The ______________________* is a "pit present" in the "center" of the ________

macula lutea	______________,* a "yellowish spot" on the retina (Fig. 7.1).
fovea centralis	**749** This ______________________* ("central pit") consists of a layer of closely packed *cone* cells, yielding the sharpest vision when light is focused upon it through the *lens* (Fig. 7.1).
membran mening -oid chor/oid (kō' roid)	**750** *Chor,* like ____________ (frame 424) and ____________ (frame 636), is a root for "membrane." And ________, the suffix in *arachnoid* (frame 640), means "like or resembling." Consequently, ________/______ translates as "resembling a membrane."
choroid retina sclera	**751** The ____________ is the black middle layer of the eyeball wall that looks "like" a dark "membrane" between the ____________ ("net") present on the inside and the "hard" ____________ forming the external layer of the eyeball wall (Fig. 7.1).
hyal aque/ous (ā' kwē əs, ak' wē əs) vitre/ous (vit' rē əs)	**752** A *humor* is a "fluid." *Aque* means "water" while *vitre,* like ________ (frame 458), stands for "glass." Both of these new roots take the adjectival suffix in *cartilaginous* (frame 426). Thus ________/______ is a complete term for "watery" and __________/______, like *hyal/ine* (frame 459), "refers to glass."
aqueous humor vitreous humor	**753** The ______________________* is a "watery fluid" located anterior to the lens, while the thicker ______________ ______,* "like" hot melted "fluid glass," lies in the chamber posterior to the lens (Fig. 7.1).

vitreous	**754** The ______________ ("glassy") *humor* presses against the hairlike structures supporting the lens. *Cili* means either "hair" or "eyelash."
-ary cili/ary (sil' ē er ē)	**755** Recall that ________, the suffix in both *pituitary* and *mammillary* (frame 662), means "characterized by." Then ________/______ is a term indicating "characterization by a hair or eyelash."
ciliary	**756** Examination of Figure 7.1 reveals that the lens is attached to the ______________ *body* by connections having the "characteristics" of the "hairs" on the "eyelashes"!
ir/is (ī' ris)	**757** If *ir* is a root for "rainbow" then ____/____ means "presence of a rainbow." In this case the suffix is that found within *femoris* (frame 584).
iris	**758** The ________ is a circular disk "present" in the eye that can be any one of several different colors of the "rainbow."
pup/il -il	**759** If *pup* is a root for "girl" or "doll" then ______ /_____ means "little girl" or "little doll," where ______, the suffix of *myofibril* (frame 552), is employed.
pupil iris	**760** The __________ ("little girl") is the contractile opening "present" at the center of the ________ ("rainbow").
	761 A girl can see herself as a "little girl" or a "lit-

pupils

tle doll" mirrored in the black ________ of the irises of someone looking directly at her, hence the strange source for this term (Fig. 7.1)!

Meat/us (mē ā' təs)

762

The pupil is simply a special type of opening. *Meat* is a root for an "opening" or a "passage" in general. ______/____ then means "presence of an opening or a passage," where the suffix of *vagus* (frame 730) is used.

---

acoustic

auditory

meatus

763

The ____________ ("referring to hearing," frame 730) or ____________ ("characterized by hearing," frame 730) ________ ("opening") is an external "passage present" in the ear (Fig. 7.2).

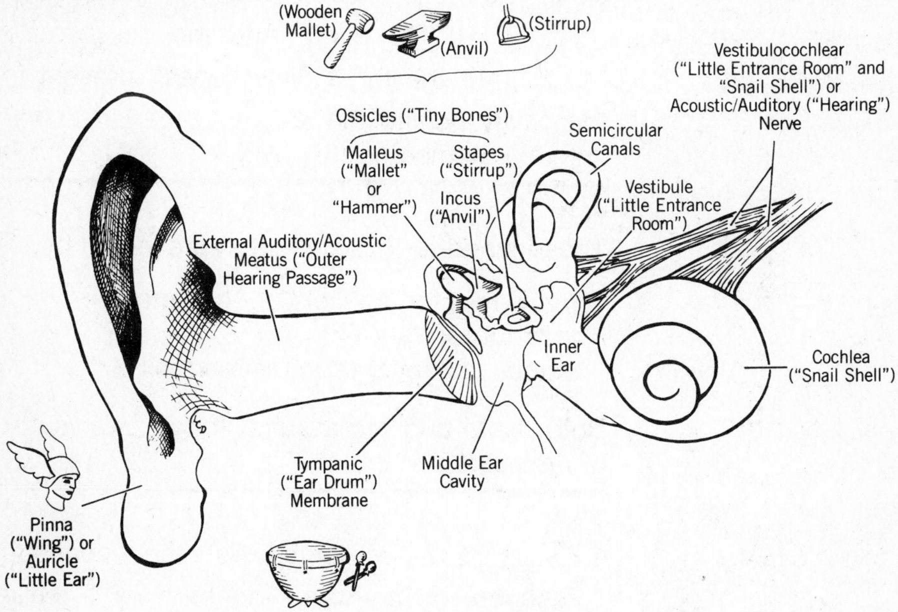

Figure 7.2. STRUCTURES OF THE EAR

---

tympan/ic

764

If *tympan* means "drum" then ____________/

(tim pan′ ik)	____ denotes "referral to a drum," where the ending of *somatic* (frame 723) is borrowed.
auditory/acoustic meatus tympanic	**765** Sound waves entering the external ______ ______________________* ("hearing passage") beat against the ____________ ("drum") *membrane.*
auric/le (ô′ ri kəl) ossic/le (os′ i kəl)	**766** If *auric* means "ear" and *ossic* means "bone," then _________/____ represents "little ear" and _________/____ represents "little bone." In each case the suffix of *peduncle* (frame 675) is assumed.
pinna auricle ossicles tympanic	**767** The external portion of the ear is thus called either the _________ ("wing") or the ______ ________ ("little ear"). And the ________ ______ are the three "tiny bones" present in the cavity behind the ____________ (ear "drum") membrane (Fig. 7.2).
-us	**768** These inner-ear ossicles are represented by: *malle* root for "mallet" or "hammer" *inc* root for "anvil" *stapes* (stā′ pēz) term for "stirrup" Both *malle* and *inc* assume the ______ suffix of *meatus.*
Malle/us (mal′ ē əs) inc/us (ing′ kəs)	**769** _________/____ embodies the concept, "presence of a mallet or hammer," while ______/____ embodies the notion of an "anvil being present."
malleus	**770** The ___________ is a "hammer/mallet"-shaped bone that moves against the ____

incus stapes cochle/a (kok′ lē ə)	_____ ("anvil"-shaped bone). This bone pushes on the _________ ("stirrup-shaped" bone), which in turn depresses the oval window of the _________/__ ("snail shell," frame 728; use suffix *-a*) (Fig. 7.2).
 retina acoustic/auditory	**771** Just as *rods* and *cones* are the visual receptors within the _________ (innermost "net" of eyeball wall), the *hair cells* are the _____________ ("hearing") receptors within the *organ of Corti* (kôr′ tē).
organ of Corti cochlea Corti	**772** The _______________________* is a spiral organ inside the _________, a "snail shell"-like structure "present" within the inner ear. This main sensory organ of hearing is named in honor of the Italian anatomist Alfonso _________ (Fig. 7.3).
    utric/le (yo͞o′ tri kəl) sacc/ule (sak′ yo͞ol)	**773** A *labyrinth* (lab′ ə rinth) is a "maze." *Utric* oddly means "skin bag." *Sacc* simply denotes a "sac." The former root uses the diminutive suffix in *ossicle*, the latter root the ending in *microtubule* (frame 233). Thus _________/_____ is "small skin bag" and _______/______ is "little sac."
     Labyrinth	**774** The *Minotaur* (min′ ə tôr) was a man-eating monster of Greek myth. This creature had the head of a bull and the body of a man! To keep the fearful beast under control it was kept in the ____________, a *maze*like prison with no escape!
labyrinth	**775** The ____________ ("maze") of the inner ear, like the mythical prison of the Minotaur, is a complex network of hollow tubes and

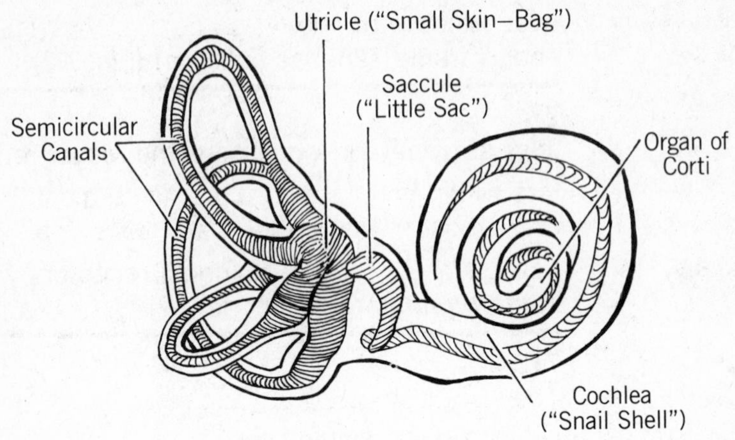

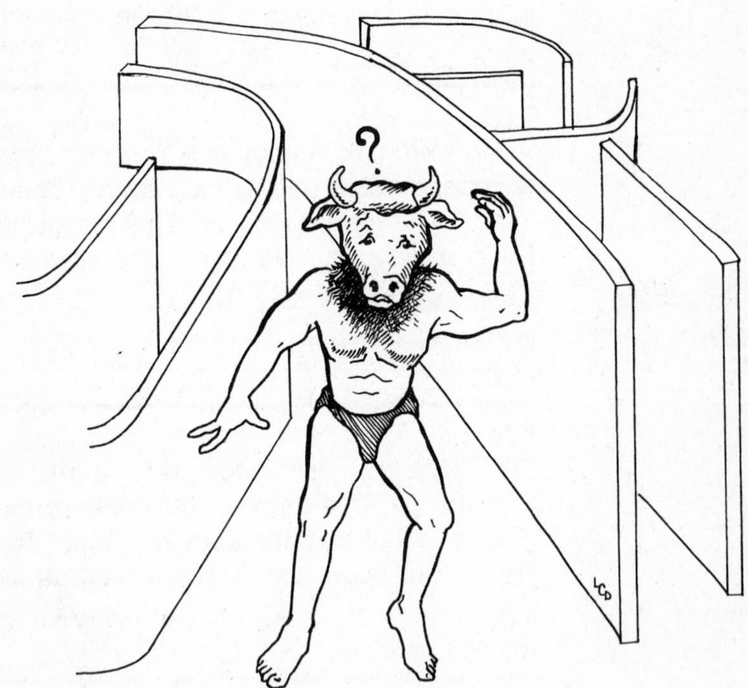

Minotaur Lost in the Labyrinth
(Prison "Maze")

Figure 7.3. THE LABYRINTH AND THE MINOTAUR

utricle saccule	passageways. Among these are the semicircular canals, the ________________ ("small skin bag"), and the ________________ ("little sac") (Fig. 7.3).
labyrinth	**776** The ________________ ("maze" of tubes) contributes to body equilibrium and balance, without which we would be as helpless and confused as the imprisoned Minotaur!

Now do the Self-Test for Unit 7 (page 275 in the Appendix).

UNIT 8
TERMS OF THE GLANDS

Answer	Frame
gland glandular	**777** Recall that ________ (frame 378) means "acorn" and that ________ (frame 380) denotes "reference to a little acorn." All such "acorns" produce secretions. *Crin/e* translates as "presence of a secretion."
Endo- exo-	**778** ________, the prefix in *endoneurium* (frame 694), like *en-* and *intra-*, means "internal." And ________ (Table 3, frame 38) like *e-, ecto-*, and *extra-*, is a prefix meaning "external."
endo/crin/e (en′ də krin) exo/crin/e (ek′ sə krin)	**779** Therefore ____/____/__ is equivalent to "presence of an internal secretion," while ____/____/__ is the counterpart meaning "presence of an external secretion."
Endocrine hormones	**780** *Hormon/e* denotes "presence of an arousal or a setting into motion." ________ glands are those which "secrete internally," releasing ________ into the bloodstream, which, when "present, arouse or set into motion" a variety of physiological responses.
Exocrine	**781** ________ glands are those which "secrete externally," releasing some useful product into a duct that carries it "out" to a body surface.

Table 8.1 ESSENTIAL TERMINOLOGY OF THE ENDOCRINE GLANDS

adrenal	estrogen	progesterone
adrenalin	exocrine	prolactin
adrenaline	glucagon	somatotrophic
adrenocorti-cotrophic	glucocorticoid	somatotropic
aldosterone	glucose	steroid
antidiuretic	hormone	testosterone
corticoid	insulin	thymus
corticotrophic	Langerhans	thyroid
cortisol	mineralo-corticoid	thyrotrophic
diuretic	oxytocin	thyroxin
endocrine	pancreas	thyroxine
epinephrine	parathyroid	trophic
		tropic

782

endocrine hormones mitosis	Just as ________ ("internally secreting") glands release minute quantities of ________ that "arouse" dramatic processes of body growth and other vital functions, a small *acorn* planted into the ground gives off roots that "set into motion" a dynamic sequence of ________ ("condition of threads," frame 340) culminating in a towering oak tree. Hence the analogy between *gland* and "acorn."

783

somat	Remember that ________ (frame 723), like *som* (frame 216), is a root for "body." The former root takes *o* as its combining vowel. Both *troph*, a root for "nourish" or "feed," and *trop*, a root for "turn" or "change," can be used with the root for "body."

784

Troph/ic (trō′ fik) trop/ic (trō′ pik)	________/____ means "nourishing or feeding," while ________/____ means "turning or changing." In each case *-ic* is an appropriate suffix.

Somat/o/troph/ic (sō′ mə tō trō′ fik) somat/o/trop/ic (sō′ mə tō trō′ pik)	**785** ______/__/______/___ is a term "pertaining to feeding the body," and ____ ____/___/_____/___ is a term for "pertaining to changing the body."
hormone pituitary hypophysis	**786** Both of the terms in frame 785 describe the same ________ ("arouser," frame 780). This chemical is secreted by the anterior portion of the _________ ("characterized by mucus," frame 662) *gland* or _____ _______ ("presence of an undergrowth," frame 662).
somatotrophic somatotropic	**787** This anterior pituitary secretion is sometimes called ____________ ("feeding the body") *hormone* or is alternately called ____________ ("changing the body") *hormone*. These two contrasting names indicate that this single hormone has a "nourishing" effect on the cells, "turning" them on and "feeding body" growth and continuous "change." Consequently, it is also called the *pituitary growth hormone*.
trophic tropic	**788** The anterior pituitary gland is the "acorn" that secretes ________ ("nourishing") or _______ ("turning" on) hormones of various kinds. For simplicity, from now on this book will use the "pertaining to nourishing" ending only.
somatotrophic	**789** Besides *somat* in ____________ ("pertaining to body nourishment"), other roots can be used with *o* plus *trophic* to name anterior pituitary hormones. Observe the list below: *ren* "kidney"

Answer	Frame
cortic	________ "cortex" or "bark" (frame 738) *thyr* "shield"
ad- ad/ren/o	**790** Recall that ______, the prefix in *adduction* (frame 571), means "toward." Thus, ____/ ______/__ represents a root and combining vowel for "toward the kidney."
Ad/ren/al (a drē′ nəl)	**791** ____/______/____ "pertains to (something) toward the kidney," where *-al*, not *-ic*, is the "pertaining to" suffix. Here no connecting vowel is necessary.
adrenal	**792** The ____________ *gland* is located "toward" or near the upper pole of the "kidney." Hence its name.
cerebrum	**793** The adrenal gland, just like the ________ ________ ("presence of main brain mass," frame 626), has an outer "bark" or *cortex*.
cortic/o/troph/ic (kôr′ ti kō trō′ fik)	**794** Referring back to frames 785 and 789, you should conclude that just as *somatotrophic* "pertains to feeding the body," __________/ __/__________/____ "pertains to nourishing the cortex."
ad/ren/o/cortic/o/troph/ic (a drē′ nō kôr′ ti kō trō′ fik)	**795** Finally, ____/______/__/____________/__/ __________/____ is a long single term that "refers to nourishing the adrenal cortex."
Adrenocorticotrophic	**796** ________________________ *hormone* from the anterior pituitary is a chemical messenger that stimulates or in a sense "nourishes" ("feeds into") the activity of the "adrenal cortex."

thyr/o/troph/ic (thī′ rō trō′ fik)	**797** *Somatotrophic* hormone and *adrenocorticotrophic* hormone are joined by a third *trophic* hormone described as ________/__/__________/____ ("pertaining to nourishing a shield;" consult frame 789).
Thyrotrophic thyr/oid (thī′ roid)	**798** ______________________ *hormone* stimulates the ________/______ ("shield-resembling;" use suffix in *choroid*, frame 750) *gland.*
thyroid	**799** Thyrotrophic hormone is also called *TSH*, where *T* is the abbreviation for ______ ________, *S* the abbreviation for *stimulating*, and *H* the abbreviation for *hormone.*
thyroid	**800** The right main lobe or left main lobe of the ______________ *gland* taken singly strikingly "resembles" the oblong "shield" of an African warrior. Taken together, the two lobes with their central connection look like the shields of two warriors pressing hands (Fig. 8.1).
cortic/oid	**801** If *thyroid* means "resembling a shield," it stands to reason that ____________/______ means "resembling a cortex." However, in this case "oid" actually refers to the presence of a *steroid* (stir′ oid, ster′ oid).
ster/oid	**802** If *ster* means "solid oil" then ________/______ denotes "solid oil resembler."
steroids lipid	**803** The ________________ ("solid oil resemblers") are a group of chemicals belonging to the __________ ("fat resembling," frame 303) family. They are all characterized by the pres-

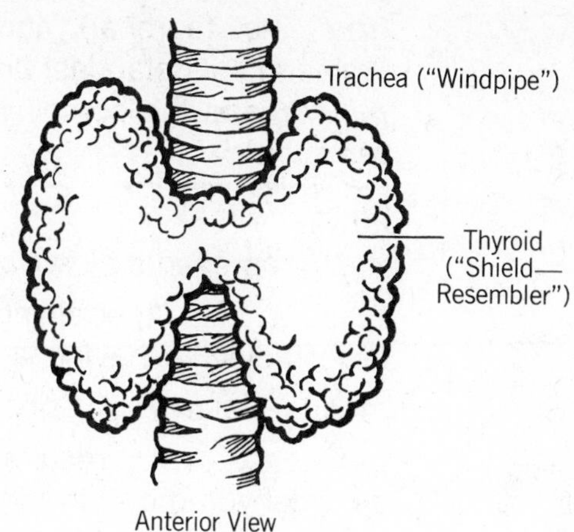

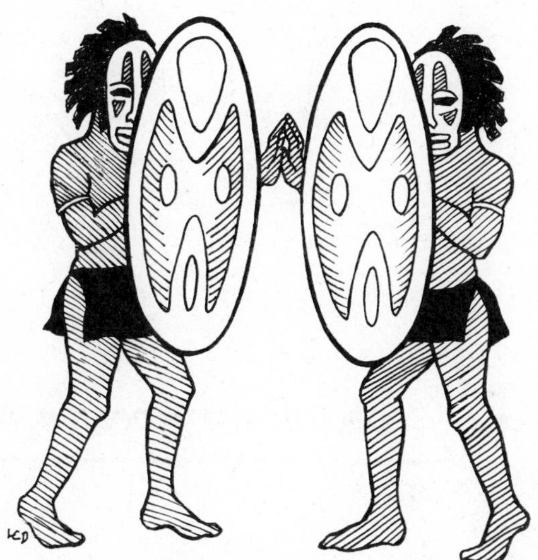

Oblong Shields of African Warriors

Figure 8.1. THE THYROID GLAND "SHIELD"

	ence of three six-carbon ring molecules attached to a single five-carbon ring molecule.
corticoid	**804** Then __________ really means "steroid from the (adrenal) cortex."
mineral/o/cortic/oid (min′ ər al o kôr′ ti koid)	**805** It is easy to assign the name of __________ ____/__/__________/______ to a "steroid

from the (adrenal) cortex" that deals with "mineral" substances! Just use the entire term *mineral* and the combining vowel within *somatotrophic*!

---

organic ald/o/sterone (al dos' tə rōn)	**806** *Ald/o* represents *aldehyde* (al' də hīd), an ____________ ("pertaining to carbon," frame 267) molecule having a -CHO group. *Sterone* means "steroid." Consequently, ______/__/ ____________ results from the addition of an aldehyde group to the steroid ring (Fig. 8.2).

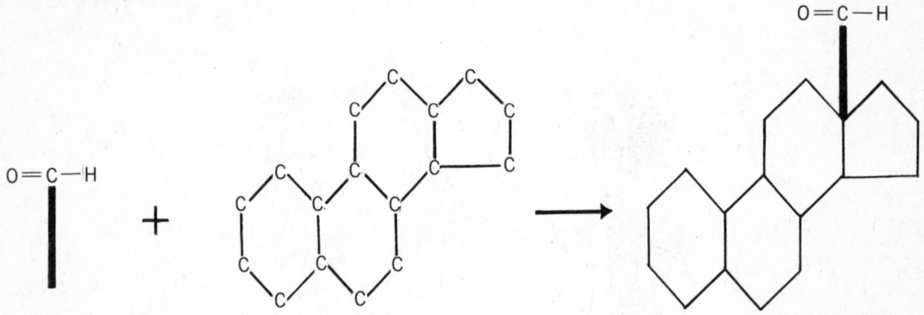

Figure 8.2. PRODUCTION OF ALDOSTERONE

Aldosterone mineralocorticoid	**807** ____________________ ("aldehyde + steroid") is the major ____________________ ____________ ("steroid mineral" regulator from the adrenal "cortex").
glyc gluc/ose	**808** *Gluc*, like ________ (frame 312), is a root for "sweet." And *-ose* is a suffix meaning "a type of sugar or other carbohydrate." Consequently, ________/______ translates as "a type of sweet sugar."
glucose	**809** You may remember ______________ as an

Answers	Frames
monosaccharide	important type of ____________ ____________ ("single sugar," frame 311) with the chemical formula $C_6H_{12}0_6$.
gluc/o/cortic/oid (glo͞o′ kō côr′ ti koid)	**810** Utilizing the appropriate root and combining vowel, we can construct ________/__/________/________ for "steroid from the (adrenal) cortex" that deals with "glucose." This term has an ending identical to that of *mineralocorticoid*.
cortic cortis/ol (kôr′ ti sol)	**811** *Cortis*, like ____________ (frame 738), is a root for "cortex." The suffix *-ol* means "alcohol" or "related to alcohol." Thus ____________/____ literally means "alcohol" (from the) "cortex."
Cortisol glucocorticoid	**812** ____________, the main ____________ ____________ ("steroid from the cortex" that handles "glucose"), is structurally "related to alcohol."
cortisol mineralocorticoids adrenocorticotrophic	**813** Both the *glucocorticoids*, such as ____________, and the ____________ ____________, such as *aldosterone*, are secreted by the adrenal cortex. But it is mainly the *glucocorticoid* family of hormones that are secreted in response to ____________ ____________ ("nourishing the adrenal cortex," frame 795) *hormone* from the anterior pituitary gland.
aldosterone	**814** Besides ____________ ("aldehyde plus steroid"), there are a number of other hormones containing the steroid ring structure and having names ending with *sterone*. *Test/o* means "eggshell" while *pro/gest* means "be-

Answer	Frame
pro-	fore bearing," where ______, the prefix in *prophase* (frame 344), means "first" or "before."
test/o/sterone (tes tos′ tə rōn) pro/gest/erone (prō jes′ tə rōn)	**815** Consequently, ______/__/______ is a "steroid" hormone secreted by paired glands in the male that resemble "eggshells." And ______/______/______ is a "steroid" secreted by the female "before bearing" a child. In this term *-erone* means the same as *-sterone*.
testosterone progesterone	**816** Not surprisingly, ______ ("eggshell steroid") is often called the "male sex hormone," while ______ ("before-bearing steroid") is often nicknamed the "pregnancy hormone."
gen Estr/o/gen (es′ trə jən)	**817** Recall that ______, the suffix in *glycogen* (frame 312), means "produce." *Estr* is a root for "mad desire," which commonly takes *o* as its combining vowel. ______/__/______ then means "mad desire producer."
Estrogen	**818** ______, often nicknamed the main "female sex hormone," is a steroid known to "produce mad desire" for sexual intercourse in nonhuman female mammals at regular intervals.
steroid	**819** You have learned that two endings, *-oid* (as in mineralocortic*oid*) and *-sterone* (as in testo*sterone*), indicate a ______ (steroid/nonsteroid) hormone structure.
-in	**820** But not all hormones are steroids! And some hormones are partly named for their acid-base nature. Remember that ______, the suffix in

	both *myosin* (frame 559) and *myelin* (frame 700), generally denotes "a neutral substance." "Basic substances" are usually indicated by the chemical suffix *-ine*. Some roots involved with *-in* or *-ine* for naming hormones are given below:
	insul "little island"
oxy	______ "swift" or "oxygen" (frame 333)
	toc "birth"
	lact "milk"
	thyrox (same as *thyr*, frame 789)
shield	"____________"
	nephr (same as *ren*, frame 789)
kidney	"____________"
	821
Thyrox/in; thyrox/ine (thī rok′ sin)	__________/____ or ___________/______ is "a neutral or basic substance" (secreted by the) "shield."
	822
Throxine; throxin	______________ or ______________ is the
thyroid	principal hormone released from the ______ ________ ("shield-resembling") *gland* in the neck.
	823
Para-	________, the prefix in *parasympathetic*
para/thyr/oid (par ə thī′ roid)	(frame 719) means "beside." Then _______/ ________/______ is interpreted as "beside the shield resembler."
	824
parathyroid	The ___________________ *glands* are four small bodies located "beside the thyroid" that secrete their own hormone involved with calcium metabolism.
	825
oxy/toc/in (ok′ sē tō′ sin)	Reviewing frame 820, build a term translatable as "a neutral substance" (that promotes) "swift birth": ______/______/____.

Oxytocin

826
_______________ is a hormone that stimulates contraction of the walls of the womb during delivery, helping to assure a "swift birth" process.

pro/lact/in
(prō lak' tin)

827
Use the prefix in *progesterone* to aid you in constructing _____/_______/____, a term that means "a neutral substance" (secreted) "before milk."

Prolactin

828
________________ must be released into the bloodstream "before milk" can be secreted from the breasts.

epi/nephr/ine
(ep i nef' rin)

829
Employ the prefix in *epineurium* (frame 692) plus information from frame 820 to help you build _____/__________/_____, which can be deciphered as "a basic substance" (from a gland) "upon the kidney."

ad/renal

ad/renal/in

ad/renal/ine
(ə dren' ə lin)

830
Perhaps you remember from frame 792 that the ____/_________ glands are those located "toward" the top of the "kidney." You can use this entire term to make either ____/_________/____ or ____/__________/_____, representing "a neutral or basic substance" (secreted by the gland) "toward the kidney."

epinephrine

adrenalin

adrenaline

831
Actually ______________________, containing the "kidney" root *nephr*, and both ________________ and ________________, containing the "kidney" root *ren*, are three different names for one single hormone!

832
Epinephrine is the more "scientific" name for

adrenaline adrenalin	this hormone, while ______________ and ______________ seem to be the more "common" or "trade" names for the chemical.
medulla cortex	**833** This hormone is secreted by the *adrenal* ______________ ("middle or marrow," frame 684) *not* by the outer *adrenal* ______________ ("bark").
insul/in (in′ syoo lin, in′ sə lin)	**834** Looking back one final time at frame 820, pick the appropriate root to synthesize __________/____, a term meaning "a neutral substance" (secreted by) "little islands."
Insulin Langerhans	**835** ______________ is a hormone secreted by "little islands" of endocrine tissue within the *pancreas*. These "little islands" are formally called the *islets of Langerhans* (läng′ ər häns) to credit their German discoverer, Paul ______________.
gluc glucose	**836** *Glucag*, like ________ (frame 808) and *glyc*, (frame 312) is a root for "sweet" that usually represents ______________ ("a type of sweet sugar," frame 808).
glucag/on (gloo′ kə gon)	**837** Borrow the suffix from *axon* (frame 696) and develop a term that indicates "presence of glucose or sweetness": ____________/____.
Glucagon	**838** ______________, like *insulin*, is secreted by the "little islands" of the pancreas. But unlike insulin, which *decreases* blood glucose, this hormone, when "present" in the bloodstream,

acts to *increase* the blood "glucose" and thereby preserve blood "sweetness"! In essence, this particular hormone helps to ensure that *glucose* is never *gone* from the bloodstream!

---

flesh; pan/creas

839
Aristotle (ar′ i stot əl), the famous Greek philosopher who studied anatomy by animal dissection, used the term *pancreas*. *Pan* is a prefix for "all," while *creas*, like *sarc* (frame 519), means "________." Thus _____/________ translates literally as "all flesh."

---

pancreas

thym/us (thī′ məs)

840
The ______________ ("all flesh") has an ancient Greek counterpart, *pankreas*, "the sweetbread." Interestingly, *thym*, a different root, also means "sweetbread" in Greek! This root takes the "presence of" suffix found within *meatus* (frame 762). Consequently, ________/____ denotes "presence of a sweetbread."

---

pancreas

thymus

glucose

841
Both ______________ ("all flesh") and ____ ________ ("sweetbread presence") are examples of "sweetbread." The "sweet" probably comes from the taste of ______________ ("a type of sweet sugar," frame 808) associated with these two glands. *Thym* enters in because the *sweet*-smelling leaves of the common garden *thyme* are used for seasoning, a fact that Aristotle and his predecessors must have used for the naming process!

842
The "bread" in "sweetbread" probably comes from Old English and means "roasted meat." Therefore "sweetbread" can be reinterpreted as "sweet roasted meat" from the *pancreas* and *thymus* gland! Aristotle analyzed living things in terms of their supposed "purposes."

pancreas

insulin

glucagon

The term ______________ or "all flesh" obviously derives from the notion that the "purpose" of this gland is to serve as "flesh" for the human dinner table! You must understand that this name was given some 2,000 years before the discovery of the important hormones ______________ ("a neutral substance" from "little islands," frame 834) and ______________ ("presence of glucose or sweetness," frame 837)!

---

thymus

843
To Aristotle and associates, the sweet delicate flavor of the roasted *pancreas* and ______________ ("sweetbread presence") must have seemed much like the spicy tang of *thyme*!

---

sternum

844
The *pancreas* is located behind the inferior edge of the stomach, while the *thymus* is a flat gland just behind the ______________ ("breast bone," frame 478) and projecting upward into the base of the neck (Fig. 8.3).

---

thymus

pancreas

845
Examination of Figure 8.3 should allow you to correctly surmise that the ______________ (pancreas/thymus) in the young calf or lamb is called the "throat sweetbread," while the ______________ (pancreas/thymus) is commonly called the "stomach sweetbread" of older calves.

---

pancreas

Anti-

846
Adequate secretion of insulin from the ______________ ("all flesh") helps to ensure that *glucose* is not normally excreted in the urine. Likewise, another hormone is "against" excessive excretion of water in the urine. ______________ (Table 4, frame 42) is a prefix for "against."

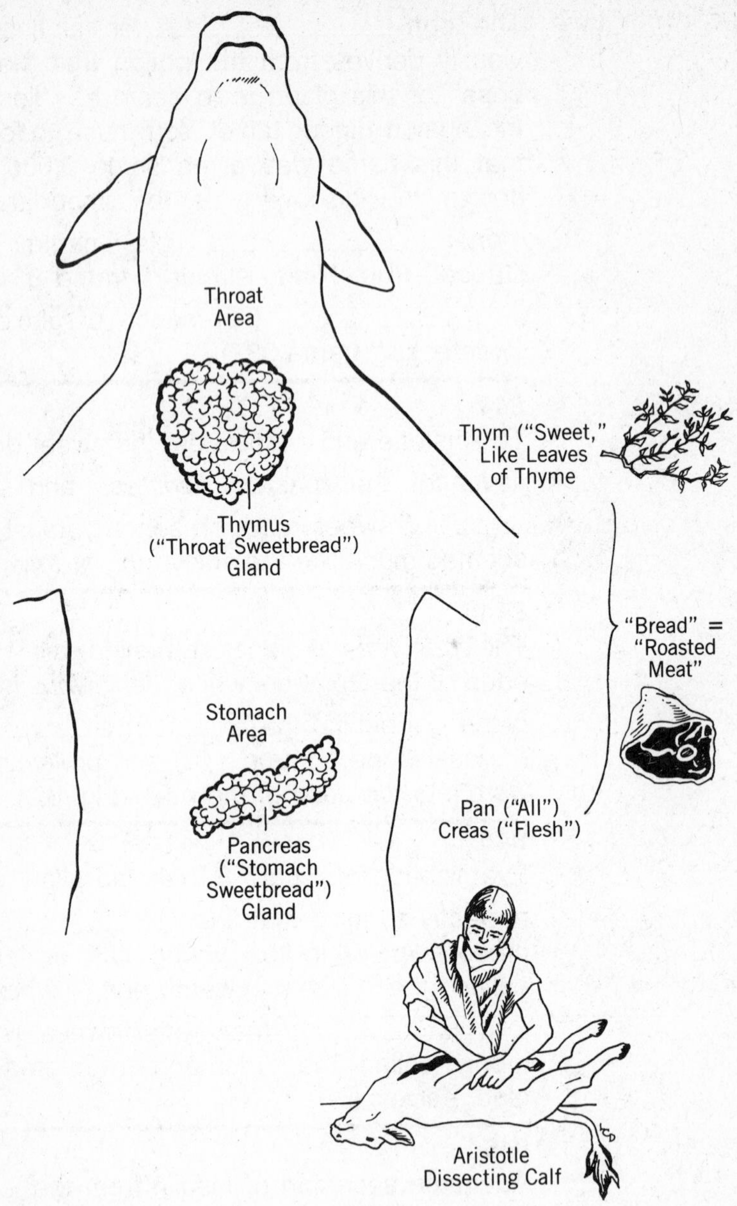

Figure 8.3. "SWEETBREADS"

847

Diuret is a root meaning "urine through." It derives from *dia* ("through") plus *urin* ("urine"). This root assumes the "pertaining to" suffix in

diuret/ic (dī yoo ret′ ik, dī ər et′ ik)	*tropic* (frame 784). As a result you can build ____________/____, a term "referring to urine (passing) through" the body.
diuretic anti/diuret/ic (an′ tē dī ər et′ ik)	**848** If ______________ "pertains to urine (passing) through" the body and being excreted, then _______/___________/_____ is a term "referring to" a process operating "against urine (passing) through" the body.
Antidiuretic hypothalamus pituitary	**849** ______________________ *hormone* is actually produced by special cells in the _______ ______________ (region "present below the bedroom," frame 654). Stored and released by the posterior portion of the _________ _______ ("characterized by phlegm," frame 662) gland, this hormone increases H_2O reabsorption into the bloodstream from the kidney tubules. This increased water reabsorption effectively opposes or works "against" excretion of large quantities of dilute "urine."

Now do the Self-Test for Unit 8 (page 276 in the Appendix).

UNIT 9
TERMS OF THE HEART AND MAJOR BLOOD VESSELS

cardi/ac	**850** The heart (*cardi*) is like an inverted two-story house (Fig. 9.1). The pointed "tip" or "peak" of the roof is represented by the heart *apex* (ā' peks). And the broad foundation of the house is similar to the __________/____ ("pertaining to the heart;" use *-ac* rather than *-ic*) *base*.
apex	**851** The great vessels, the major *arteries* and *veins*, enter or leave the heart at its *base*, much like plumbing or gas pipes connect to the house foundation (Fig. 9.1). The ________ ("pointed tip") lacks any such connections.
Cardi/um	**852** __________/____ designates "presence of the heart" just as *neur/i/um* (frame 691) indicates "presence of a nerve."
pericardium (per i kär' dē əm)	**853** And ____________________ is a loose-fitting sac "present around the heart" in the same way that *perineurium* (frame 693) is "present around nerve" fascicles.
epicardium (ep i kär' dē əm)	**854** The ____________________ lies "upon the heart" like a thin coat of paint. Similarly, the

Table 9.1 TERMS OF THE HEART AND ASSOCIATED VESSELS

aorta	diastolic	systole
aortic	endocardium	systolic
apex	endothelium	tricuspid
artery	epicardium	tunica adventitia
arteries	inferior vena cava	tunica externa
arterioles		tunica interna
atria	lumen	tunica intima
atrial	mitral	tunica media
atrioventricular	myocardium	tunicas
atrium	pericardium	vasoconstriction
A-V	pulmonary	vasodilation
bicuspid	S-A	vena cava
capillary	semilunar	venous
capillaries	sinoatrial	ventricular
cardiac	sinus	venules
cardium	superior vena cava	
diastole		

epineurium (frame 692) is "present upon nerve."

---

myocardium (mī′ ō kär′ dē əm)

855
Using *my/o*, we can say that the ________________ is the actual "muscle present" in the "heart" wall (Fig. 9.1).

---

auricle

856
The heart has both a right ________ ("little ear," frame 766) and a left one, which project out from the heart surface like awnings from exterior windows (Fig. 9.1).

---

aort/a (ā ôr′ tə)

857
If *aort* means "lifting up," then ________/__ means "presence of a lifting up," where the suffix of *cochlea* (frame 770) is employed.

---

coronoid

coron/ary (kôr′ ə ner ē)

858
Recall from frame 475 that ________________ is translated as "crownlike." Using the suffix in *mammillary* (frame 662), build ________/______ ("characterized by a crown").

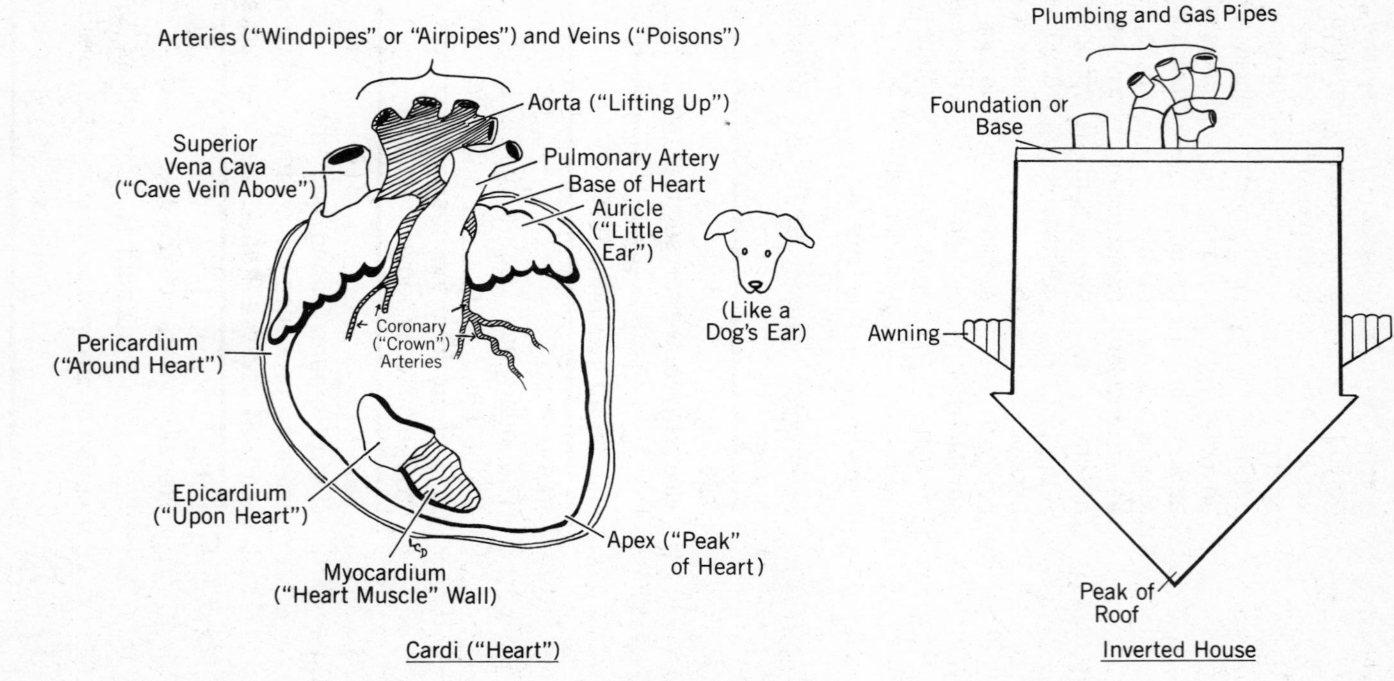

Figure 9.1. **HEART AND HOUSE: EXTERIOR FRONTAL VIEW**

aorta
coronary
auricles

859
The ___ ______ is the main artery "present" at the base of the heart. It "lifts up" the blood out of the heart to serve most of the body. The ________________ arteries arise from the bottom of this main artery and encircle the heart with all the essential "characteristics of a crown" that has slipped down over a prince's ________________ ("little ears") (Fig. 9.1).

arter/y
-y

860
If *arter* means "windpipe," then __________/ __ is the simple term for the "condition of being a windpipe." In this case the ____ ending of *anatomy* (frame 70) is assumed.

Artery

861
______________ ("windpipe condition") is actually a misnomer. The name was coined several thousand years ago, and it indicates that the ancient anatomists were convinced these hollow "pipes" contained "wind" (air) rather than blood!

arter/ies

862
Singular terms ending in *-y* generally form plurals using *-ies*. For example __________/ ______ represents "more than one artery."

arteries

863
The ________________ ("windpipes or airpipes") contract after death and blood stagnates in the veins, leaving these "pipes" empty except for "air."

artery
lumen

864
Lumen (lo͞o′ mən, lyo͞o′ mən) is an entire term from the Latin for "light space." Upon cutting open an ____________ ("airpipe condition") of a slain enemy soldier, the early scholars probably observed an empty __________ or

	"space" that allowed room "light" to penetrate deep into the vessel interior.
lumen	**865** Since the arteries carry no blood and have an empty ________ ("light space") after death, it was not unreasonable for early thinkers to assume that they were merely "airpipes" connecting each "lung" (*pulmon*) to the central "windpipe" in the chest.
Pulmon/ary (pool′ mə ner ē, pul′ mə ner ē)	**866** __________/______ means "characterized by the lung" just as *coronary* is "characterized by a crown."
pulmonary	**867** The right ________________ artery is "characterized by" the fact that it carries oxygen-poor blood from the heart to the right "lung." This blood is blue, like that in a coronary "vein" (*ven*).
Ven ven/ous (vē′ nəs)	**868** _____ (the root for "vein") means "poison," as in the deadly *venom* of a striking rattlesnake! And ______/______ "pertains to poison or a vein," much as *vitreous* (frame 752) "pertains to glass."
Venous	**869** __________ blood leaving most organs contains the "poisonous" waste products of body cells.
arter/i/oles (är tir′ ē ōlz) ven/ules (ven′ yo͞olz)	**870** Since *centr/i/oles* (frame 230) are "tiny centers," _________/__/_______ must be "tiny arteries." Likewise, if *tub/ules* (frame 233) are "small tubes," then ______/_______ are "small veins."

Answer	Frame
capill/ary (kap′ i ler ē)	**871** *Capill* is Latin for "hair." *Coronary* is to *coron* as ______/____ is to *capill.*
Capillaries arterioles venules	**872** ________ are tiny blood vessels "characterized by" a slender appearance much like short "hairs." These minute hairlike vessels branch off from larger ________ ("tiny arteries") feeding into a tissue. The poisonous waste products from the tissue eventually enter the ________ ("small veins").
Cav/a (kā′ və)	**873** Groups of *venules* collect into larger *veins.* Two major veins are so big that they are named with *cav* ("cave"). ____/__ denotes "presence of a cave," just as *ven/a* (vē′ nə) means "presence of a vein."
vena cava inferior vena cava	**874** The *superior* ________* ("presence of a cave vein") and the ________* ("cave vein present below") are two huge *veins* that, like large *caves* filled with dark slow-moving water, return blue venous blood to the right upper chamber of the heart.
atri/um (ā′ trē əm)	**875** If *atri* is a "room" or "entrance room," then ____/__ denotes "presence of an entrance room," where the suffix is the same as that in *epicardium.*
endo/cardi/um (en do kär′ dē əm)	**876** And ____/____/__ represents something "present within the heart" just as *endoneurium* (frame 694) represents something "present within nerve."

endocardium atrium	**877** A frontal section through the heart, with the anterior portion removed, reveals an ________________ or lining "present within the heart" chambers. Each upper chamber serves as an ____________ or "entrance room present" at the top to receive blood flowing into the heart from the large veins (Fig. 9.2).
atri/a (ā' trē ə)	**878** Terms whose singular forms end in *-um* usually form plurals with *-a*. Consequently, ________/__ represents "more than one atrium."
atria ventricles	**879** If the heart is an *inverted* two-story house, then the __________ form the "rooms" upstairs while the ____________________ ("little bellies," frame 657) are the rooms downstairs (Fig. 9.2).
ventricul/ar (ven trik' yə lər)	**880** Even though *ventricle* is an entire term for "little belly," *ventricul* is only a root with the same meaning. We can add the suffix of *vestibulocochlear* (frame 730) to this root and build ________________/____ ("pertaining to a little belly").
atri/o/ventricul/ar (ā' trē ō ven trik' yə lər)	**881** *A-V* is a common abbreviation for ________/__/__________________/____, a single term for "pertaining to rooms and little bellies," whose two roots are connected by an *o* combining vowel.
atrioventricular atria ventricles	**882** The ________________________________ or *A-V* valves are like doors that open only one way: from the __________ (upper "entrance rooms") into the ________________ beneath (Fig. 9.2).

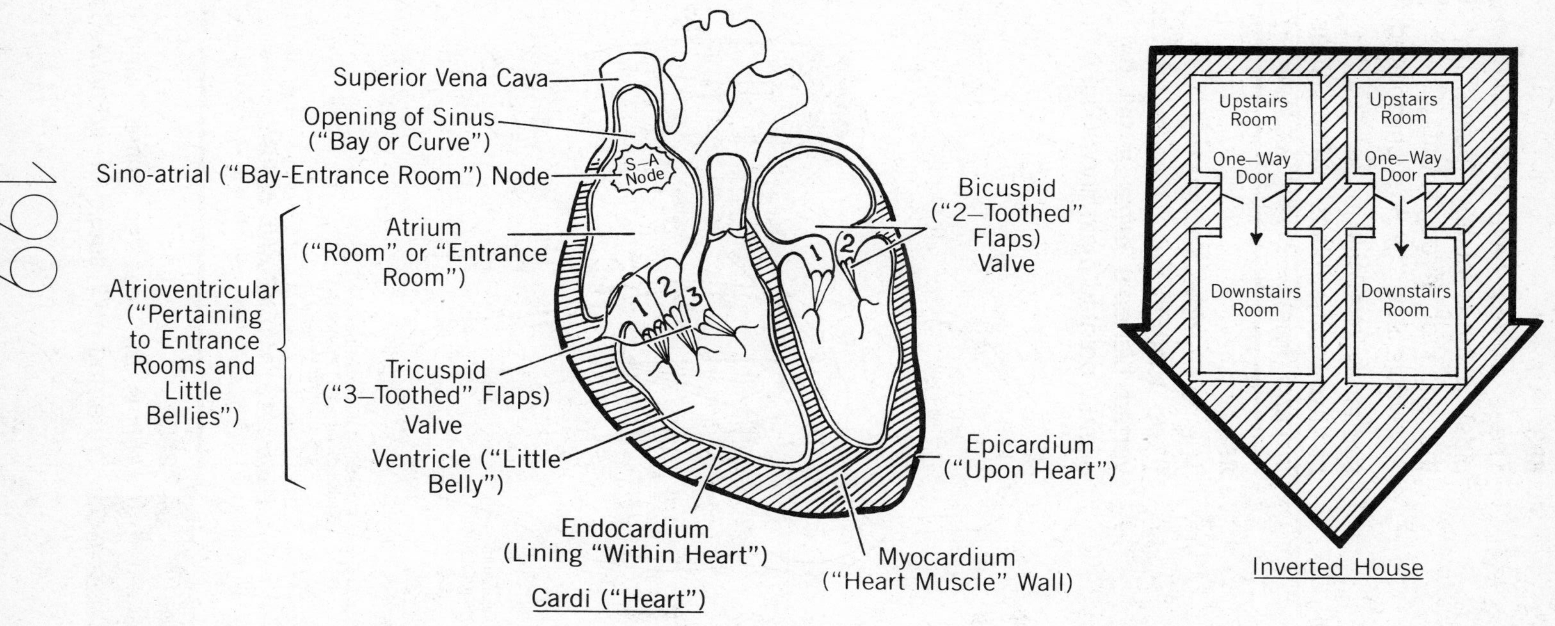

Figure 9.2. HEART AND HOUSE: INTERIOR FRONTAL VIEW

883

These valves have flaps with *cuspids* (kus pids), a fringe of tiny "points" or "teeth" like the edge of a rough leaf (Fig. 9.2). The left A-V valve has "two" such pointed flaps. Consequently, we call it the ____/________ or "two toothed flaps" valve just as we call the *bi/ceps* (frame 591) a "two headed" muscle!

bi/cuspid (bī kus' pid)

884

The *left atrioventricular* or __________ ("two toothed flaps") *valve* resembles an inverted bishop's *mitre*, a tall hat having two slightly pointed main flaps (Fig. 9.3).

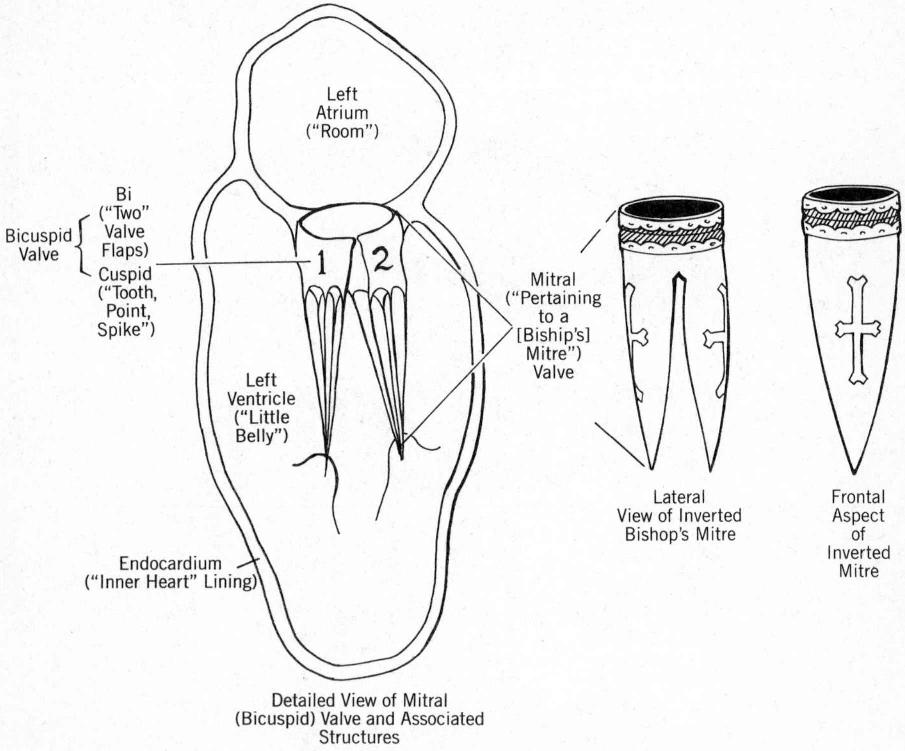

bicuspid

Figure 9.3. VALVE AND MITRE

885

Mitr is the root for "mitre," and it takes the "referring to" suffix of *adrenal* (frame 791).

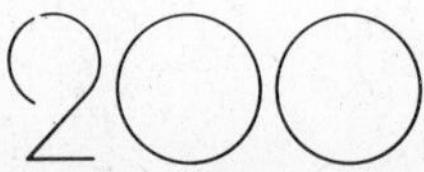

mitr/al (mī′ trəl)	Therefore ________/____ "pertains to a mitre."
A-V bicuspid mitral	**886** The valve separating the left atrium from the left ventricle is thus known by the three names of *left* ______ (atrioventricular), ________ ______ ("two toothed flaps"), or ________ ____ ("referring to a mitre") *valve*.
tri/cuspid (trī kus′ pid)	**887** The *right A-V valve* is also called the ______/ ____________ *valve* because it has "three toothed flaps," just as the *triceps* muscle (frame 591) has "three heads" (Fig. 9.2)!
sin	**888** *Sinus* (sī′ nəs) is a term containing the root ______, which means "curve" or "bay." The suffix is identical to the one seen in *thymus* (frame 840).
superior vena cava sinus venous	**889** The terminal end of the ________________ ________________* ("cave vein above," frame 874) is like a huge __________ or "bay present" near the top of the heart that "curves" into the right atrium. Of course this "bay" is filled with dark ____________ ("poisonous," frame 868) blood rather than water (Fig. 9.2)!
atri/al (ā′ trē əl)	**890** *Sin* takes the combining vowel *o* and _______/ ____ means "pertaining to an entrance room" the same way that *mitr/al* means "pertaining to a bishop's mitre."
sin/o/atri/al (sī′ nō ā′ trē əl)	**891** Therefore, ______/__/________/____ is a compound word that "refers to a bay and an entrance room."

sinoatrial tricuspid	**892** When we "refer" to the __________ _____ *node* we mean a small group of specialized excitatory cells above the _____ ________ ("three toothed flaps") *valve* and near the opening of the "bay" (*superior vena cava*) in the right "entrance room." (Consult Fig. 9.2 one last time.)
sinoatrial relaxation (lengthening)	**893** After the ______________ (abbreviated as *S-A*) *node* fires, both of the atria soon contract. *Systol* is a root for "contraction" whereas *diastol* is a root meaning "_________ ______," the exact opposite.
Systol/e (sis′ tə lē) systol/ic (sis tol′ ik)	**894** _________/__ denotes "presence of a contraction" and _________/___ "pertains to a contraction" just as *scop/e* (frame 346) denotes "presence of an examination" and *scop/ic* (frame 409) "pertains to an examination."
diastol/e (dī as′ tə lē) diastol/ic (dī′ əs tol′ ik)	**895** In a similar fashion, __________/__ is the term representing "presence of relaxation" while __________/___ "refers to relaxation."
S-A systole diastole	**896** After the ____ (abbreviation for *sinoatrial*) *node* or "pacemaker" fires, a wave of excitation results in atrial __________ ("presence of contraction"). After cardiac contraction ceases a state of __________ or "relaxation" is once again "present."
Systolic ventricular	**897** __________ (Systolic/Diastolic) blood pressure is the higher pressure measured in the arteries during ____________

diastolic

("pertaining to little bellies," frame 880) contraction. Conversely, ________________ (systolic/diastolic) blood pressure is the lower pressure exerted on the walls of arteries when the large inferior heart chambers are relaxed.

---

semi/lun/ar
(sem ē lo͞o′ nər,
sem ē lyo͞o′ nər)

898

Recall that the prefix in *semipermeable* (frame 292) means either "partial" or "half." *Lun* is the root for "moon," and it takes the "pertaining to" ending found in *ventricular*. Use these facts to help build ________/________/____ ("referring to a half moon").

---

semilunar

899

There are two ________________ ("half-moon") *valves* present in the heart. They are named for the resemblance of their valve flaps to "half moons" in the evening sky (Fig. 9.4).

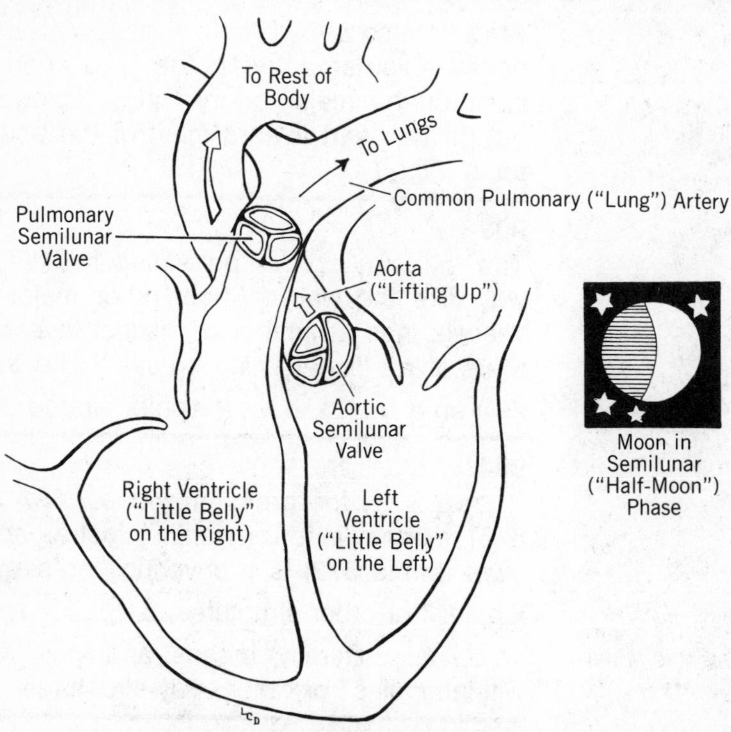

Figure 9.4. SEMILUNAR VALVES

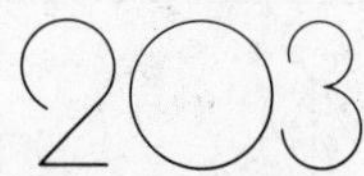

Answers	Frame
pulmonary aort	**900** Both of these valves are pushed open by the force of ventricular systole. But they differ in several ways. Recall that ________________ (frame 866) is "characterized by the lungs." And ________, the root for "lifting up" (frame 857) combines with the adjectival suffix in *diastolic*.
semilunar pulmonary	**901** The *right* ________________ ("partial moon") *valve* is "characterized by" its location at the base of the *common* ________________ *artery*, which sends blood out of the heart towards the "lungs" (Fig. 9.4).
semilunar aort/ic	**902** The *left* ________________ ("half moon") *valve* is also called the ________/____ *valve* because its name "refers to" its location at the base of the major artery "lifting" blood "up" out of the heart toward most of the body systems (Fig. 9.4).
aortic theli	**903** The ____________ ("pertaining to lifting up") wall, like the wall of most other major blood vessels, has a number of distinct layers. First, there is an "inner lining present" like the soft skin on a __________ ("nipple," frame 371).
Endo- endo/theli/um (en dō thē′ lē əm)	**904** __________, the prefix in *endocardium* (frame 876), means "inner or within." Just as *epi/theli/um* (frame 372) is a covering "present upon nipples" or other structures, ________/________/____ literally means a lining "present within nipples" or other body structures.
endothelium	**905** Blood vessels have an "inner" lining or ________________ (epithelium/endo-

lumen

thelium) "present." This deepest lining makes direct contact with the vessel __________ ("light space," frame 864) (Fig. 9.5).

---

tunicas

906

Tunic/a (tyo͞o′ ni kə, to͞o′ ni kə) denotes "presence of a coat or sheath." Originally it represented a garment worn by both sexes in ancient Greece and Rome (Fig. 9.5). Observe and pronounce the list of three different ____ __________ or "coats present" below:

tunica interna or *intima* (in′ ti mə)
tunica media
tunica externa or *adventitia* (ad ven tish′ ē ə)

---

tunica externa/ adventitia

tunica interna/ intima

tunica media

907

Using your best intuition and your knowledge of the meanings of previous terms like *internal* and *external* (both in frame 80) and *medial* (frame 154), try to correctly identify each of the different *tunicas* in this narration: "The __________ ______________________* is the 'outer coat,' which appears to be 'going out toward an adventure' with the connective tissue immediately surrounding the vessel. The ______________________* is the 'inner coat,' which makes close 'intimate' contact with the endothelium of the vessel wall. Finally the ______________________* is the 'middle' muscular 'coat' of the vessel wall" (Fig. 9.5).

---

endothelium

tunicas

908

Just as the ______________________ ("presence within nipple") can be compared to the naked skin of a citizen of ancient Rome, so the ______________ ("coats") of blood vessels are like the expensive garments that invested Caesar's royal body!

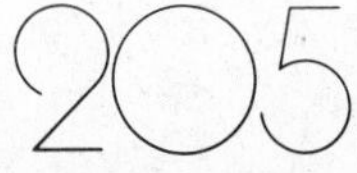

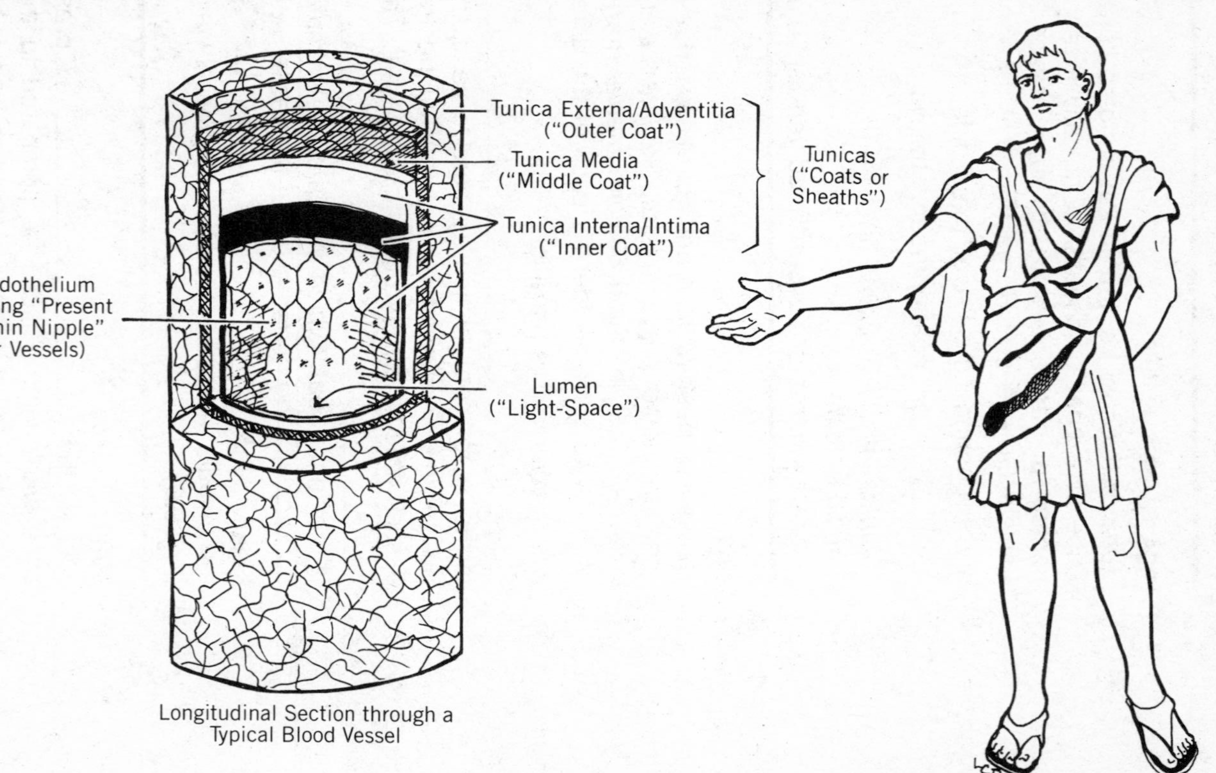

Figure 9.5. BLOOD VESSEL AND TUNICS

909

Constriction is "the act of narrowing," where ________, a suffix also found within *extension* (frame 571), means "the act or process of." *Vas/o* (vas' ō) is a root plus combining vowel for a "vessel" in general. Consequently, ______/ __/________________/______ can be built as a term meaning "the process of vessel narrowing."

-ion

vas/o/constrict/ion

910

Dilat means "widen." Thus ______/__/______ ____/______ translates as "the process of vessel widening."

vas/o/dilat/ion
(vas' ō dī lā' shən)

911

______________________________ (Vasoconstriction/Vasodilation) of arterioles occurs when the smooth muscle of the __________ ______________* ("middle coat present") contracts and "acts to narrow the vessel" lumen. __________________________ (Vasoconstriction/Vasodilation) results when the smooth muscle present in this middle sheath relaxes, "acting to widen the vessel" lumen.

Vasoconstriction

tunica media

Vasodilation

Now do the Self-Test for Unit 9 (page 278 in the Appendix).

UNIT 10
TERMS OF THE BLOOD AND LYMPHATIC SYSTEM

Answer	Frame
cardi vas cardi/o/vascul/ar (kär′ dē ō vas′ kyə lər)	**912** From study of Unit 9 you should know that ________/o means "heart" and that ______ (frame 909) is a root for "vessel." Similarly, *vascul* is a root meaning "little vessel," which can take the same suffix as *semilunar* (frame 898). As a result ________/__/ ________/____"refers to the heart and little vessels."
cardiovascular	**913** The ________________________ *system* is one that "pertains to the heart" and all the blood "vessels," both large and "small."
matter cytoplasm plasma	**914** *Plasm/a* (plaz′ mə) denotes "presence of ____________" (frame 191). Just as ____ ______________ (frame 194) is the fluid "matter" within the "cell," ____________ is the fluid "matter present" within the bloodstream.
Cyt	**915** ______ (frame 190), the root for "cell" in *cytoplasm*, can combine with suffix *-e* at the end of a term. The following word parts can be used with this format to indicate the kind or nature of the cell in question:

Table 10.1 TERMS OF THE BLOOD AND LYMPH

acidophil	erythrocyte	lymphocyte
agglutination	fibrin	lymphopoiesis
agglutinin	fibrinogen	monocyte
agglutinogen	globulin	neutrophil
albumin	hematopoiesis	plasma
antibodies	hemoglobin	prothrombin
antigen	immunity	reticulo-endothelial
basophil	leukocyte	thrombin
cardiovascular	lymph	thrombocyte
eosin	lymphatic	
eosinophil		

erythr/o (i rith′ rō) "red"
leuk/o (lyo͞o kō or lo͞o′ rō) "white"
__________ "single" (frame 310)
lymph/o (lim′ fō) "clear spring water"
thromb/o (throm′ bō) "clot"

mono-

916

In addition to the __________ or fluid "matter," name these cell types also "present" in the blood:

"__________ is a general term for 'white' blood 'cell.' Literally translated from the Latin, __________ is a specific type of white blood 'cell' also found in 'clear spring water.' And a __________ is another type of white 'cell' having a 'single' large horseshoe-shaped nucleus.

An __________ is simply a 'red cell' in the blood, while a __________ is a small 'cell' fragment involved with 'clot' formation."

plasma
Leukocyte
lymphocyte
monocyte
erythrocyte
thrombocyte

917

Some particular __________ or "white cells present" in the blood are named for their apparent "love" (*phil*) for certain biological tissue stains. These cellular stains enhance visibility of structures seen through the microscope. Observe and pronounce the following cell types:

leukocytes

neutrophil (nyo͞o′ trə fil)
basophil (bas′ ə fil, bā sə fil)
acidophil (a sid′ ə fil)
eosinophil (ē ō sin′ ə fil)

---

bas/o/phil

acid/o/phil

neutr/o/phil

918
Obviously, a ______/__/____________ has a "love" or chemical affinity for "basic" dyes whereas the ________/__/________ is well demonstrated using "acidic" dyes. And ______ ____/__/________ clearly describes a cell that "loves neutral" chemical stains only!

Eosin (ē′ ə sin)

919
__________, one of the two roots in *eosinophil*, comes from the Greek for "dawn." It is an acidic stain that is pink like the rose-colored "dawn."

---

eosin/o/phil

920
The striking pink appearance of the ____ ______/__/________ under the microscope does indeed suggest that it "loves" the rose-colored sky at "dawn"!

---

condition of being

921
Immun comes from the Latin for "exempt," as in being free or "exempt" from disease. According to Table 8 (frame 55) *-ity* is a suffix meaning "______________________________ ______."*

---

immun/ity
(i myo͞o′ ni tē)

922
Thus you can build __________/______ for a "condition of being exempt."

---

leukocytes

immunity

923
Most of the different ______________ ("white cells") play crucial roles in __________ ______, that is, our "condition of being exempt" from disease.

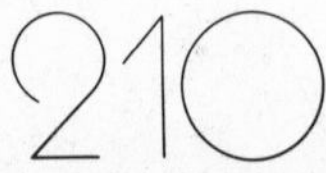

Reticul endo/theli/al	**924** ______/ o (frame 197) means "little network," while ______/______/____ (frame 904) refers to (something) within nipples," where *-al* is the appropriate suffix.
Reticul/o/endo/theli/al (re tik' yə lō en dō thē' lē əl)	**925** ______/__/______/______/____ is a single long term that "pertains to a little network" of defensive cells located as a lining "within" the inner walls of some vessels and organs.
monocyte reticuloendothelial phagocytosis	**926** For example, the ______, a white "cell" with a "single" prominent nucleus, is often considered a member of the ______ ______ ("little network within nipples") *system*. This is because it engages in ______ ("condition of cell eating," frame 300) of foreign cells and debris, thereby aiding in body defense.
anti/gen (an' ti jən)	**927** The prefix in *antidiuretic* (frame 848) combines with the ending in *estrogen* (frame 817) to make ______/______, a foreign substance that stimulates the body to "produce" defensive chemicals that act "against" it.
antibodies	**928** These defensive chemicals are called ____ ______ because they literally represent the response of the "body against" harmful assault!
antigens erythrocytes	**929** For example, there are chemical ______ ______ present on the surfaces of ______ ______ ("red cells") that may

antibodies	cause ______________ to be "produced against" them in the "body" of another person not having these chemical markers.

930

	To cite a specific instance, let us say that a large quantity of type A blood is transfused into a type B individual. The type A person's
antigen	erythrocytes all carry the A __________ (antibody/antigen). The type B individual's
antibodies	blood serum contains *anti-A* __________ ______ (antibodies/antigens). The attack of these defensive "body" chemicals "produced against" the foreign red cells is called an *antigen-antibody reaction* (Fig. 10.1).

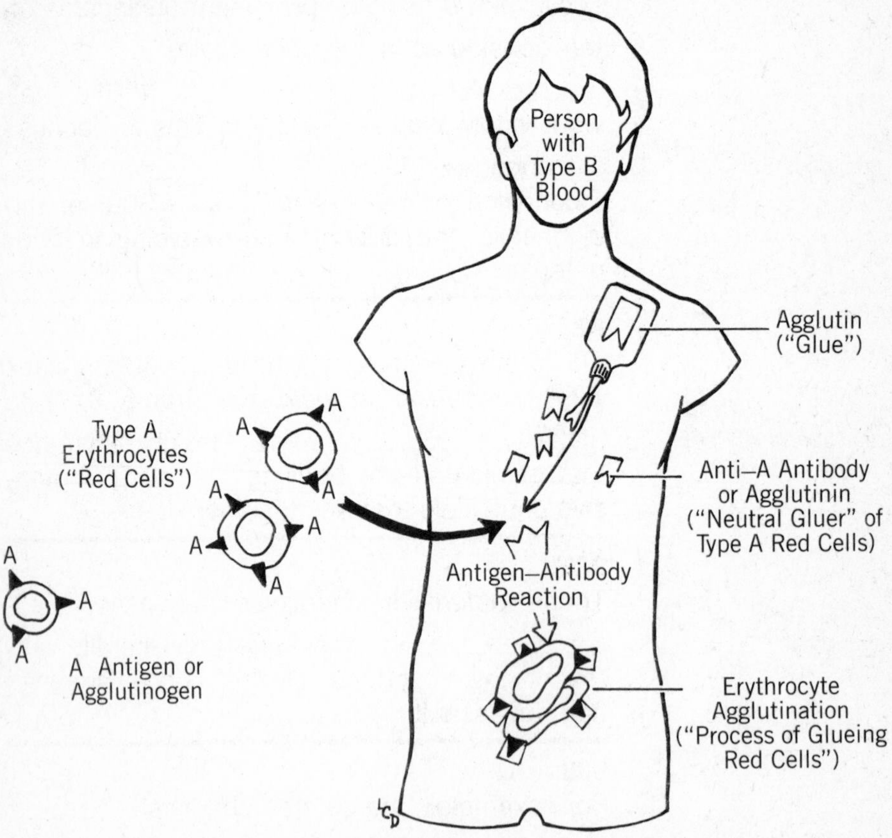

Figure 10.1. BLOOD ANTIGENS AND ANTIBODIES

Answer	Frame
agglutin/in (ə glo͞o′ tə nin)	**931** If *agglutin* is a root for "glue," then ______________/____ is a term for "neutral substance that glues." In this case, the suffix is the same as that in *insulin* (frame 834).
agglutinin	**932** An ________________ is simply a "neutral" *antibody* that "glues" or clumps together red blood cells bearing a foreign *antigen* (Fig. 10.1).
agglutin/o/gen (ag lo͞o tin′ ə jən, ə glo͞o′ tə nə jən)	**933** Using the same root, the combining vowel *o*, and the suffix of *antigen*, build ____________/__/______ ("gluing producer").
agglutinogen	**934** An ________________ is simply an *antigen* that stimulates the body to "produce gluing" or clumping of the foreign erythrocytes carrying it (Fig. 10.1).
agglutinogen agglutinin	**935** An ________________ (agglutinin/agglutinogen) is a special type of *antigen*, while an ________________ (agglutinin/agglutinogen) is a special type of *antibody*.
-gen	**936** The fact that both *antigen* and *agglutinogen* in frame 935 end with ________ may help you to remember that they both mean about the same thing.
agglutin agglutinat/ion (ə glo͞o tə nā′ shən)	**937** *Agglutinat* like ________________ (frame 931) is a root for "glue." Using the suffix of *vasodilation* (frame 910), build ____________/______, a term meaning "the process of gluing."

Agglutination agglutinins agglutinogens	**938** ________________ is the potentially dangerous "process of gluing" or clumping together of foreign red cells in a patient. This process is due to the action of his/her ________________ ("neutral substances that glue," frame 931) on the ________________ ("gluing producers," frame 933) attached to these incompatible transfused erythrocytes (Fig. 10.1).
lymph lymphocytes	**939** Antibodies are found in the ________ ("clear spring water," frame 915) as well as in the blood. In fact, certain ____________ ("clear spring water cells," frame 916) change into cells that directly produce the antibodies!
glob -in	**940** The following word parts are used in naming blood proteins, some of which can function as antibodies: *globul* "little globe" ________ "globe" *hem/o* "blood" *album* "egg white" Several of these roots take _____, the suffix for "neutral substance."
Hem/o/glob/in (hē′ mə glō bin) globul/in (glob′ yə lin) album/in (al byo͞o′ min)	**941** _____/__/_______/____ is a "neutral globe in the blood." A __________/____ is a "neutral little globe." And __________/____ is a "neutral egg white substance."
Albumins	**942** ______________, a group of proteins in raw "egg white," are also present in the human

osmosis
Hemoglobin
globulins

blood plasma, where they affect ______________ ("condition of thrusting," frame 296). ______________ is a "globe"-shaped protein located within the red "blood" cell. And ______________ are a group of plasma proteins shaped like "small globes," some of which function as antibodies.

Lymph/o/poiesis
(lim′ fō poi ē′ sis)

943
The suffix *-poiesis* means "formation of (something)." ________/__/__________ is "formation of clear spring water," where *o* is the appropriate connector.

---

hem
hemat/o/poiesis
(hem′ ə tō poi ē′ sis)

944
Hemat, like ________, means "blood," and ________/__/__________ is "formation of blood," just as the term in frame 943 is "formation of lymph."

Lymphopoiesis
capillaries
Hematopoiesis

945
______________ or "formation of lymph" largely occurs because of the leaking of "clear spring water" out of tiny blood ______________ ("characterized by hairs," frame 872). ______________ or "formation of blood" is largely a function of the bone marrow.

Lymphat
Lymphat/ic
(lim fat′ ik)

946
________, like *lymph*, is a root for "clear spring water" in the same manner that *hemat,* like *hem*, is a root for "blood." ________/____ "pertains to lymph," where *-ic* is the suffix.

---

lymphatic

947
The phrase ______________ *system* "refers to" the vessels and organs that collect and modify the fluid strikingly resembling "clear spring water."

---

thromb/in

thromb

948
The lymphatic system is not directly involved in the process of blood clotting. But a number of plasma proteins are! Using frame 940 as an example, we can construct __________/ ____ as a "neutral clotting substance," where __________, the root for "clot" (frame 915), is employed.

pro/thromb/in
(prō throm′ bin)

949
And borrowing the prefix of *prolactin* (frame 827), you can build ______/__________/ ____ ("before a neutral clotting substance").

Prothrombin

thrombin

950
__________________ is the inactive protein that exists first, "before" being converted into the active "clotting" enzyme __________ ______.

fibr

fibr/in

951
Recall that ________, the root in *fibril* (frame 551), means "fiber." Thus ________/____ is a "neutral fiber substance."

fibr/in/o/gen
(fī brin′ ə jən)

952
This "neutral fiber substance" term can connect with the suffix of *agglutinogen* (frame 933) using a bridging *o* to result in: ________/ ______/___/______.

Thrombin

fibrinogen

fibrin

953
______________ ("neutral clotting substance") acts upon ________________ ("neutral fiber producer"), changing it into __________ ("neutral fiber").

fibrin

954
The __________ ("neutral fiber substance") actually consists of whitish protein filaments

that interlace to form the blood clot plugging a hole in a severed vessel.

---

thrombocytes

955
This meshwork of tiny whitish fibrin filaments catches passing ______________ ("clot cells," frame 916) in the bloodstream like fish in a taut sticky net. These "clot cells" are really just "little plates" or *platelets* (plāt′ ləts) of cell fragments.

Now do the Self-Test for Unit 10 (page 279 in the Appendix.)

UNIT 11
TERMS OF THE RESPIRATORY SYSTEM

sternum thoracic	**956** Pretend you have x-ray eyes! Use them to zoom in on the middle of the human ______________ ("chest presence," frame 476). Your vision pierces right through the associated bone and nearby ribs, directly into the ______________ ("referring to chest," frame 100) *cavity*.
pleur/a (ploor' ə)	**957** If *pleur* means "rib" or "side," then __________/__ denotes "presence of a rib" or "presence of a side." Here the suffix is that found in *tunica* (frame 906).
parietal visceral parietal pleura visceral pleura	**958** Recall from frame 83 that ______________ "refers to a wall" and ______________ "pertains to internal organs." Use this recollection to help you name the ______________ ______________,* the serous membrane lining the chest "wall" on the inner "sides" of the "ribs." Likewise, we refer to the ______________* as the membrane on the "sides" of the "internal organs" called the *lungs*.
visceral pleura	**959** From frame 958 you would judge that it is the ______________* (parietal

Table 11.1 TERMS OF RESPIRATION AND ACID-BASE BALANCE

acid	cricoid	oxyhemoglobin
acidosis	epiglottis	parietal pleura
alkali	expiration	pharyngeal
alkalosis	glottis	pharynx
alveolar	Hippocrates	pleura
alveoli	hyperventilation	respiration
alveolus	hypoventilation	respiratory
bronchi	inspiration	trachea
bronchioles	laryngeal	ventilation
bronchus	larynx	visceral pleura
carbon dioxide	mediastinum	

pleura/visceral pleura) that directly covers the surfaces of the lungs.

---

parietal pleura

960
Once your gaze has sliced through the ______________* (parietal pleura/visceral pleura) lining the wall of the chest cage, you will view the "middle" of the thoracic cavity, in the region internal to the "breastplate." This region is called the *mediastinum* (mē dē əs tī′ nəm).

---

middle

sternum

961
Take an educated guess! *Media* probably means "__________," while *stinum* is almost identical to the bone called the __________.

---

mediastinum

962
The ______________ is the "mid"-region of the thoracic cavity visceral to the "sternum."

Trache/a

963
Glancing upward you can see the *trachea* (trā′ kē ə) ascending into the base of the *larynx* (lar′ ingks). __________/__ has the same "presence of" suffix as *plasma* (frame 914).

---

trachea larynx	**964** If __________ denotes "presence of a rough artery or windpipe," then __________ must logically be a complete Greek term for "upper windpipe" owing to its location superior to this structure (Fig. 11.1).
artery trachea	**965** "Wind" or air does indeed blow through these "pipes" during breathing, unlike an __________ ("condition of being a windpipe," frame 860), which in reality carries blood. The __________ or "rough artery" is made "rough" by the presence of partial rings of cartilage along its length.
larynx cartilaginous	**966** The __________ ("upper windpipe") also is largely __________ ("pertaining to cartilage," frame 426) in nature.
larynge/al (la rin′ jē əl)	**967** The root for *larynx* is *laryng* or *larynge*. Combining the latter root with the suffix of *reticulo-endothelial* (frame 925) results in __________ /____.
pharynge pharynge/al (fa rin′ jē əl)	**968** In an identical manner, *pharyng* or __________ (frame 728), the root for *pharynx* (far′ ingks), is in __________/______ ("pertaining to the throat of the windpipe").
laryngeal pharyngeal	**969** The __________ ("referring to upper windpipe") cartilages form a box for the vocal cords just below the __________ ("referring to the throat of the windpipe") passageway (Fig. 11.1).
thyr	**970** If *cric* means "ring" and ________ (frame 798)

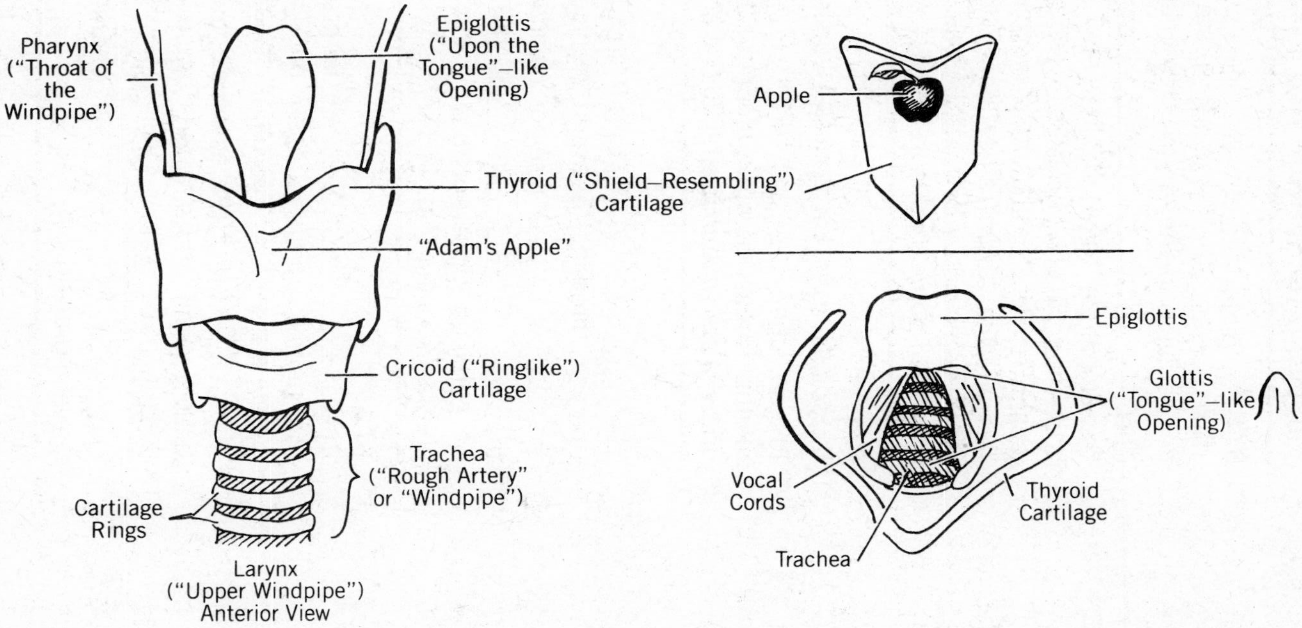

Figure 11.1. THE LARYNX

cric/oid (krī′ koid) thyr/oid	is "shield," then ________/______ means "ringlike" just as ________/______ (frame 798) means "shieldlike."

---

cricoid thyroid	**971** The ______________ *cartilage*, the most inferior cartilage of the larynx, "resembles a ring." The ______________ *cartilage*, named for its "resemblance to a shield," has an anterior projection called the *Adam's apple*. This projection is more prominent in males, hence the reference to *Adam* rather than *Eve*! It is as if *Adam*, tempted by Eve, still had a chunk of the forbidden *apple* lodged in his neck (Fig. 11.1)!

---

epi/glott/is (ep i glot′ is)	**972** If *glott/is* (glot′ is) denotes "presence of a tongue," then __________/__________/____ means "presence upon a tongue," where the prefix of *epicardium* (frame 854) is affixed.

---

glottis larynx epiglottis	**973** The ______________ is a "tongue"-shaped opening "present" between the vocal cords in the ____________ ("upper windpipe"). And the ____________________ is the leaflike lid of cartilage "present upon" this "tongue"-shaped opening (Fig. 11.1).

---

epiglottis -ory re/spirat/ory (res′ pi rə tôr ē)	**974** The ____________________ lid present "upon the glottis" remains open during breathing. *Spirat* is a root for "breathe." It combines with ________, the "characterized by" suffix in both *auditory* and *olfactory* (frame 730). *Re-* is a prefix for "back" or "again." Thus ____/ ___________/______ "is characterized by breathing again."

---

respiratory	**975** The ______________________ *system* is "characterized by" cycles of "breathing" that

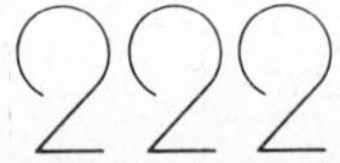

occur not once but rather happen "again." Soon after one *in*hales one starts to *ex*hale.

Re/spirat/ion (res pi rā' shən)
In/spirat/ion (in spi rā' shən)
ex/pirat/ion (eks pi rā' shən)

976
____/____________/______ is literally "the act of breathing again," where the suffix of *agglutination* (frame 937) is included. ____/____________/______ ("the act of breathing in") is soon followed by ____/__________/______ ("the act of breathing out"). Then this cycle is *re*peated "again."

---

expiration
inspiration

977
Note that the initial *s* has been dropped from the root for "breathe" in ______________ ("the process of exhaling") but that it has been retained in ______________ ("the process of inhaling").

---

ventilat/ion (ven ti lā' shən)

978
If *ventilat* means "to fan or blow" then ______________/______ is "the act of fanning or blowing."

Ventilation
respiratory

979
______________________ is "the act of blowing" air into and out of what has been called the ______________________ *tree*, a complex arrangement of branching tubes that is "characterized by breathing again" function.

---

bronch/us (brong' kəs)

980
Hippocrates (hi pok' rə tēz), an ancient Greek physician who lived around 400 B.C., is generally regarded as the "Father of Modern Medicine." It is known that he used *bronch*, a root for "windpipe," in the term ____________/____ ("presence of a windpipe"), where the suffix is the same as that in *sinus* (frame 888).

981
Bronchi (brong' kī) is the plural of ______

Answers	Frames
bronchus colliculus	________ just as *colliculi* ("little hills") is the plural of ________ (frame 670).
alveol/i (al vē′ ə lī)	**982** Similarly, if *alveol/us* (al vē′ ə ləs) denotes "presence of a tiny cavity," then ________/__ denotes "presence of tiny cavities."
bronch/i/oles (brong′ kē ōlz)	**983** And ________/__/________ are "little bronchi" just as *arter/i/oles* (frame 870) are "little arteries."
bronchi trachea bronchioles alveoli	**984** Assembling the separate pieces of this respiratory puzzle, we can say that the ________ are the two main branches of the "windpipe" trunk. These two large branches of the ________ ("rough artery or windpipe," frame 964) subdivide into many "little windpipes" or ________. Microscopic ducts in turn bud off from these "little windpipes" and terminate in clusters of ________ ("tiny cavities"), like hollow stems attaching pitted olives to the swaying branches of an inverted olive tree (Fig. 11.2).
Hippocrates respiratory alveoli	**985** We can speculate that ________ (the "Father of modern medicine") and his students might have made some mental connection between an olive tree and the ________ ("back-breathing") *tree*. But the microscopic ________, "tiny cavities" surrounded by thin walls, would certainly not have been accessible to his view!
respiration	**986** Nor would Hippocrates have known that it is actually the *alveolus*, not the *bronchus*, that is the site of ________ ("process of breathing again," frame 976).

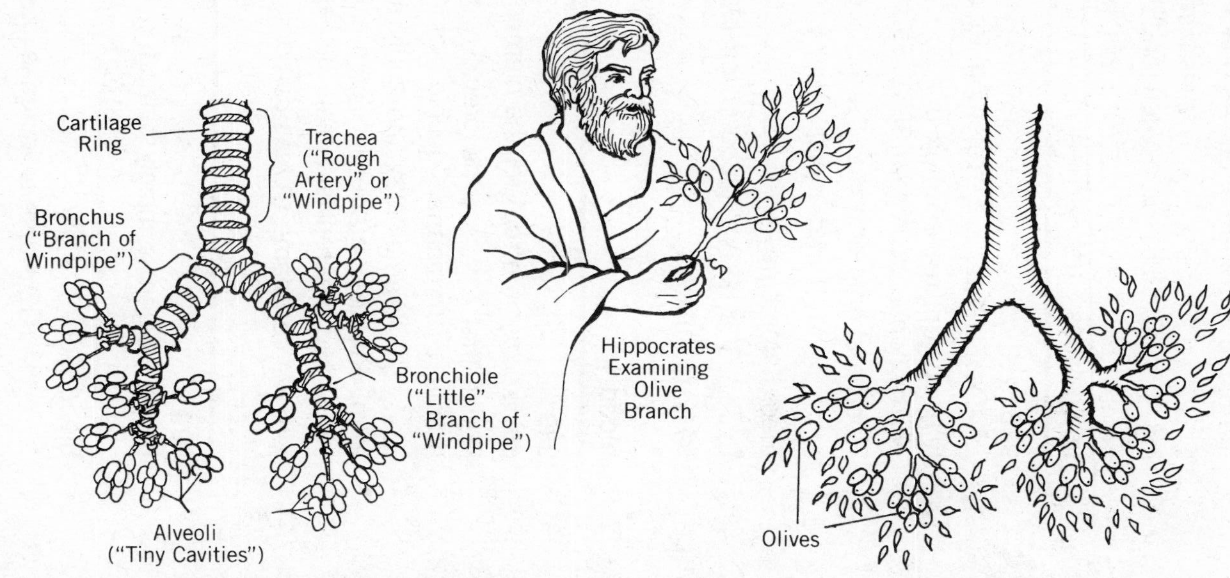

Figure 11.2. "TREES"

	987
Diffusion alveol/ar (al vē′ ə lər)	Respiration, in the sense of "breathing" gases "back" and forth "again" and again between the blood and the air, occurs only in the alveoli. ________ ("presence of scattering," frame 295) of oxygen and CO_2 occurs across the ______/____ ("pertaining to tiny cavities;" use *-ar*) wall.
	988
Alveolar oxy erythrocytes hemoglobin oxy/hem/o/glob/in (ok′ sē hē′ mə glō bin)	________ ("referring to a tiny cavity") oxygen, represented by ______ (a root in *deoxyribonucleic*, frame 335), diffuses into the blood and enters the ________ ________ ("red cells," frame 916). Once there it combines with ________ ______ ("a neutral globe in the blood," frame 941) to make ______/______/__/______/____ ("a neutral globe with oxygen in the blood").
	989
di- -ide di/ox/ide	*Ox* like *oxy* is a root for the element "oxygen." Recall that ______, the prefix in *disaccharide* (frame 310) means "double" or "two." And ________ (frame 302), the suffix in the same term, denotes "a chemical compound consisting of two different elements or parts." Therefore we can name CO_2 as *carbon* ____/____/______.
	990
oxyhemoglobin carbon dioxide	Blood oxygen is mainly carried in the form of ________ (oxygen + blood globin), while ________ ______* (CO_2) acts to increase the blood acid level.
	991
	Acid means "sour" in Latin. *Alkali* (al′ kə lī) ul-

alkali	timately derives from Arabic and means "ashes of saltwort," a type of plant that grows in places with *basic* soil. Thus a base or ________ (acid/alkali) is essentially one and the same thing.
acid alkali	**992** An ________ is a chemical with a "sour" taste that reacts with a *base* or ________ ("ashes of saltwort") to form a salt.
Acid/osis (as i dō′ sis) alkal/osis (al kə lō′ sis)	**993** ________/________ is an "acid condition" just as *arthrosis* (frame 463) is a "joint condition." And ________/________ is an "alkali condition," where the terminal *i* is dropped.
ventilation hypo/ventilat/ion hyper/ventilat/ion	**994** The prefix in *hypoglossal* (frame 730) means "below" or "deficient," while the prefix in *hypertonic* (frame 290) has the exactly opposite meaning. Combining these word parts with ________ ("the act of blowing," frame 979) we get ________/________/________ ("the act of deficient blowing") and ________/________/________ ("the act of excessive blowing").
alkalosis hyperventilation acidosis hypoventilation	**995** Respiratory ________ is a "condition of" too much body "base" due to ________, the "excessive blowing" off of too much CO_2. Conversely, respiratory ________ is a "condition of" too much body "acid" due to ________, "deficient blowing" off of CO_2.

Now do the Self-Test for Unit 11 (page 279 in the Appendix).

UNIT 12
TERMS OF THE DIGESTIVE SYSTEM

Answers	Frame
nutri aliment/ary (al i men′ tər ē)	**996** *Aliment*, like ________ (frame 515), means "nourish." Thus ____________/______ is "characterized by nourishment" just as *capillary* (frame 871) is "characterized by hair."
Saliv/ary (sal′ i ver ē) aliment	**997** *Saliv* means "saliva" or "spit." ________/______ is to *saliv* as *alimentary* is to ________.
alimentary oral salivary	**998** The ____________ ("nourishing") *tract* begins with the ______ ("pertaining to mouth," frame 104) *cavity* and its ________ ("characterized by spit") *glands*.
tongue masset	**999** *Lingu*, like *glott* (frame 972) and *gloss* (frame 728), is a root for "__________." *Mandibul* denotes "little chewer," like ________ (frame 604) represents "chew." The prefix in *subarachnoid* (frame 642) means "beneath."
Sub/lingu/al (sub ling′ gwəl) Sub/mandibul/ar (sub man dib′ yə lər)	**1000** ______/________/____ "refers to (something) beneath the tongue," where *-al* is the suffix. ______/____________/____ "refers to (something) beneath the little chewer," where *-ar* not *-al* is the appropriate ending.

Table 12.1 DIGESTIVE AND SPLENIC TERMINOLOGY

alimentary	jejunum	rugae
amylase	lipase	saliva
anus	mesentery	salivary
appendix	mucosa	serosa
cecum	muscularis	sigmoid
colon	omentum	splenic
duodenum	parotid	sublingual
esophagus	peristalsis	submandibular
gastric	peritoneum	submucosa
gastrointestinal	protease	vermiform
hepatic	pylorus	villi
hepatica	rectum	villus
ileum	ruga	

1001

Analyze *parotid* (pa rot′ id). Use your previous knowledge and your intuition. The prefix in this term is ________ ("beside"), like the prefix in *parathyroid* (frame 823). ____ ("ear"), the root, has the same meaning as *auric* (frame 766), but is closer in word structure to *ossic* ("bone," frame 766). The suffix in *lipid* (frame 303) means "belonging to a group."

par-
Ot

1002

______/_____/_____ can literally be translated as "belonging to a group beside the ear."

Par/ot/id

1003

Although the ______________ *gland* does indeed lie "beside the ear," the other two members "belonging" to the salivary gland "group" lie in more inferior locations. For example, the ____________________ *gland* hides "beneath the tongue," while the ______________ ________ *gland* rests "beneath the little chewer" or lower jaw.

parotid
sublingual
submandibular

1004

The ____________ ("spit") contains enzymes that digest or "split" apart carbohydrates. Re-

saliva

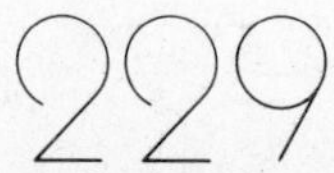

-ase lip	call (frame 319) that ________ is a suffix for "splitter." Consider these roots for chemicals: *prote* "protein" ______ "fat" (frame 303) *amyl* "starch"
 prote/ase (prō′ tē ās) lip/ase (lip′ ās) amyl/ase (am′ i lās)	**1005** A __________/______ is a "protein splitter," a ______/______ (frame 320) is a "fat splitter," and ________/______ is a "starch splitter."
  amylase lipase protease	**1006** In the digestion of a ham sandwich, the "starchy" component of the bread would be digested by ______________, while the "fat" trim of the ham would be chemically attacked by ____________ and the muscular "protein" meat itself would be digested with the aid of ________________.
 alimentary ring	**1007** A number of roots for ________________ ("nourishing") structures can add the suffix of *alveolus* (frame 982). These are: *esophag* "gullet" *pylor* "gatekeeper" *an* "________" (same meaning as *cric*, frame 970)
 esophag/us (i sof′ ə gəs) pharynx esophagus phag	**1008** The ______________/____ is the "gullet" or food-carrying tube "present" between the ____________ ("throat of the windpipe," frame 968) and the stomach. You use the ________________ ("gullet presence") when you eat. Note that the root includes ________, a root for "eat" (as found in *phagocytosis*, frame 300).

Answers	Frame
pylor/us (pī lō′ rəs) an/us (ā′ nəs)	**1009** The ________/____ is the "gatekeeper present" at the lower stomach before the small intestine, while the ____/____ is the "ring present" at the terminal end of the alimentary canal.
pylorus anus	**1010** Actually both these structures in a sense form "rings" or *sphincters* (sfingk′ tərz), ringlike bands of muscle fibers that constrict openings. The ____________ acts as a "gatekeeper," either closing or opening the "gate" between the stomach and the small intestine. And the ______ can close like a tight little "ring" to prevent release of feces from the bowel.
flank rect	**1011** Some intestinal roots using the same suffix as *ilium* (frame 128) are listed as: *duoden* "12 at a time" *jejun* "empty" or "fasting" *ile* "________" (same as for *ili*, frame 110) *cec* "blind" ______ "vertical" or "straight" (frame 600)
duoden/um (dyo͞o ō dē′ nəm) jejun/um (ji jo͞o′ nəm) ile/um (il′ ē əm)	**1012** The __________/____ is that portion of the small intestine about "12" finger-breadths in length, reflecting the crude measuring techniques of the ancient anatomists! And perhaps the ________/____ of some "fasting" subject was examined, so that the early scholars considered it "empty"! During this human dissection the ______/____ or terminal portion of the small intestine was seen "present" in the "flank"!
cec/um (sē′ kəm)	**1013** The ______/_____ is a "blind" pouch "present" at the beginning of the *colon* (kō′ lən) or

rect/um	"large intestine," and the ________/____ is a "straight" tube "present" at the end of the *colon*.
gastr/o/intestin/al (gas′ trō in tes′ ti nəl)	**1014** *Gastr* is the root for "stomach." If *intestin/al* "pertains to the intestine," then ________/ __/______________/____ "pertains to the stomach and the intestine," where *o* is the combining vowel.
gastrointestinal cecum	**1015** The ______________________ (*GI*) *system* includes the *appendix*, a thin tubular structure "appended" to the ________ ("blind" or "dead-end" pouch). This tube "resembles a worm."
-form -oid	**1016** *Vermi* is Latin for "worm" and *sigm* denotes capital "S." Recall that both ______, a suffix in *pisiform* (frame 485), and ______, the suffix in *ethmoid* (frame 480), mean "like" or "resembling."
vermi/form (vûr′ mi fôrm) sigm/oid (sig′ moid)	**1017** Thus *pisiform* is to the "pea" as ________/ ________ is to the "worm"! And *ethmoid* is to the "sieve" as ________/______ is to "S"!
vermiform appendix sigmoid colon	**1018** The ______________________ ______* is a "wormlike attachment" to the bottom of the cecum, while the ______ ______________* is the "S-shaped" portion of the "large intestine" (Fig. 12.1).
Gastr	**1019** ________, the root for "stomach," as well as *splen* ("spleen") and *hepat* ("liver") form their "pertaining to" endings with the suffix in *lymphatic* (frame 946). Consequently, we have

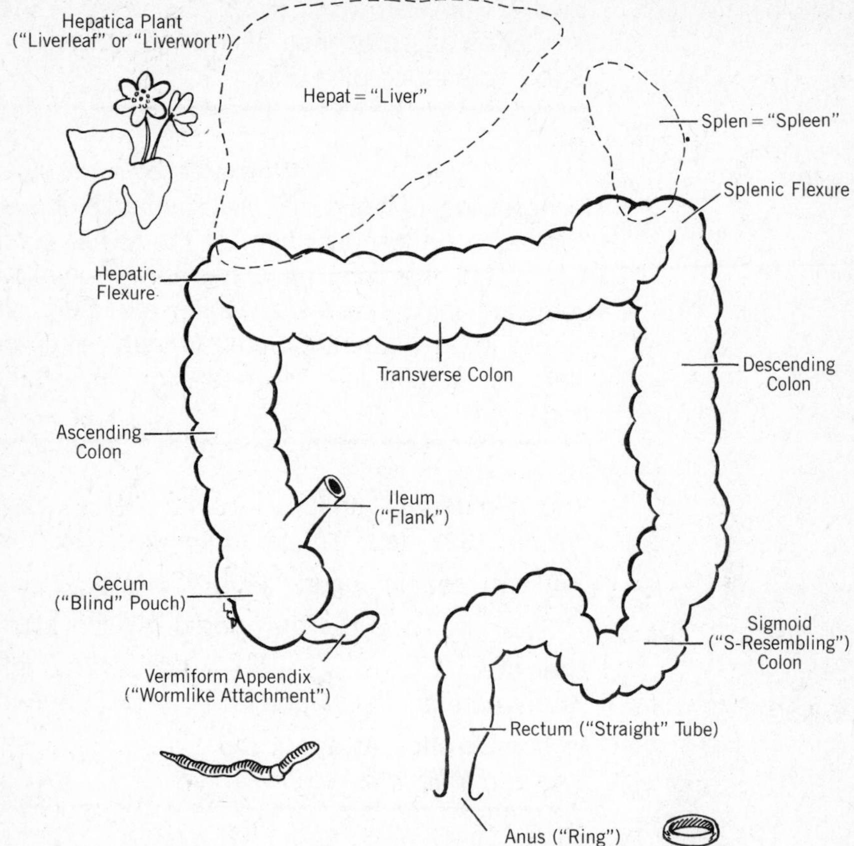

Figure 12.1. THE COLON AND ITS NEIGHBORS

gastr/ic (gas' trik) hepat/ic (hi pat' ik) splen/ic (splen' ik)	________/____ ("pertaining to the stomach"), ________/____ ("referring to the liver"), and ________/____ ("having to do with the spleen").
Gastric splenic	**1020** __________ ("stomach") function assists the process of digestion, but __________ ("spleen") function is circulatory in nature.
Hepatic	**1021** __________ means "pertaining to liver," where *hepat* is the root for "liver." But sometimes this entire term can serve as a root for

hepatic/a (hi pat′ i kə)	"liver"! For example, ______/_____ translates as "presence of the liver," where *-a* is the "presence of" suffix.

1022

Hepatica	______ is the name of a group of low-growing plants with "liver"-shaped leaves "present" on the dark floor of the forest. Each leaf of the flowering plant has three lobes resembling miniature *livers*, which turn purplish-brown in the autumn! Small wonder that the plant is also called "liverleaf" or "liverwort" (Fig. 12.1)!

1023

transverse	You might recall that ______ (frame 132) denotes "a turning across." As you can see in Figure 12.1, the ______
transverse	______ *colon* is that portion which starts
hepatic	after the ______ ("liver") *flexure* and
splenic	"turns across" the abdomen in a horizontal direction. It ends at about the ______ ("spleen") *flexure*.

1024

peri/stalsis (per i stäl′ sis)	If *stalsis* means "constriction," then ______/______ means "constriction around," where the prefix of *pericardium* (frame 853) is employed.

1025

Peristalsis	______ or "constriction around" large segments of the colon wall results in progressive movement of the feces to-
anus	ward the ______ ("ring"), like toothpaste squeezed in its tube.

1026

Here are the names of the different parts of the alimentary tract wall:

serosa (si rō′ sə)
muscularis (mus kyə lair′ is)

Answers	Frame
	mucosa (myo͞o kō′ sə) *submucosa* (sub myo͞o kō′ sə)
muscular/is peristalsis seros/a mucos/a sub/mucos/a	Of these four, it must be the ________ ______/____ that is the contracting "muscular" portion "present," resulting in ________ ______________ or "constriction around" the lumen of the digestive tube. The __________ / __ must be the "serous" membrane "present" on the outer aspect of the alimentary tract wall. The __________/__ is logically the "mucous" membrane "present" as an inner lining for the tube. Finally, the ______/__________/ __ is clearly the layer "present below" the "mucous" membrane, actually deeper in the tube wall.

Answers	Frame
serosa	**1027** Examples of ____________ ("serous" membrane) include the *peritoneum* (per i tə nē′ əm) *omentum* (ō men′ təm) *mesentery* (mes′ ən ter ē)

Answers	Frame
mes/enter/y	**1028** If *enter* is a root for "intestine" then ______/ __________/__ is the term in frame 1027 that means "condition of the middle of the intestine." (Refer back to frames 625 and 860 if necessary.)

Answers	Frame
ton peri/ton/e/um Oment/um	**1029** If *oment* is "fat skin" and ______ (frame 285) is a root for "strength, tension, or stretch," then ________/______/__/____ is the term in frame 1027 that denotes "presence of a stretching around (something)." __________/ ____ simply denotes "presence of a fat skin." In each term the suffix of *endothelium* (frame 904) is seen.

1030

The *visceral* ______________ is the serous membrane "present" within the abdominal cavity that "stretches around" and over the organs. The ______________ is a fanlike "condition of" the serosa that can be seen in the "middle" of the gap between the folds of small "intestine." And the *greater* ______________ is a serosa "present" at the inferior edge of the stomach, hanging down and covering the intestines like a "fat skin."

peritoneum

mesentery

omentum

1031

Like the *serosa*, the ______________ ("mucous" membrane) lining the digestive tube has a number of different structural modifications. Two roots for these modifications are

rug "______________" (about the same meaning as *sulc*, frame 633)

vill "tuft of hair"

mucosa

wrinkle (ditch, furrow, etc.)

1032

________/____ indicates "presence of a tuft of hair," where the suffix of *alveolus* (frame 982) is employed. ________/__ means "tufts of hair" just as *alveoli* are "tiny cavities."

Vill/us (vil′ əs)

Vill/i (vil′ ī)

1033

______/__ translates as "presence of a wrinkle" like *mucosa* (frame 1026) translates as "presence of mucus."

Rug/a (ro͞o′ gə)

1034

Terms whose singular ends with *-a* generally form plurals using *-ae*. Thus ______/______ like *sulci* (frame 635) are "wrinkles."

rug/ae (ro͞o′ jē)

1035

The mucosa of the small intestine appears to be covered with ________ ("tufts of hair")

villi

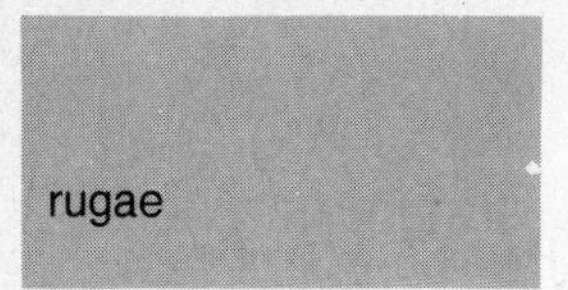

that help increase surface area for nutrient absorption. And the mucosa of the stomach is thrown into folds or __________ ("wrinkles") that have a similar function.

Now do the Self-Test for Unit 12 (page 280 in the Appendix).

UNIT 13
TERMS OF THE GENITOURINARY SYSTEM

ren nephr	**1036** Recall that both ______ (the root in *adrenal*, frame 791) and ________ (the root in *epinephrine*, frame 829) mean "kidney."
nephr/on (nef' ron) col/on	**1037** Using the latter root, build ________/____ ("presence of the kidney") just as you could have built ______/____ ("presence of the large intestine," frame 1013). In either case the suffix is that found in *mitochondrion* (frame 245).
nephron -us glomerulus (glō mer' yə ləs)	**1038** The ____________ is the primary structural and functional unit "present" in the "kidney." Each of these units is associated with a *glomerul* ("a little ball of yarn") + ______ (suffix of *anus*, frame 1009) = ______________ ("presence of a little ball of yarn").
glomerulus capillaries Bowman	**1039** The ________________ is in reality a rounded cluster of blood ____________ ("characterized by hairs," frame 872). It sits like "a little ball of (red) yarn present" in the notch of *Bowman's capsule*. This is a C-shaped chamber named in honor of Sir William __________, its discoverer (Fig. 13.1).

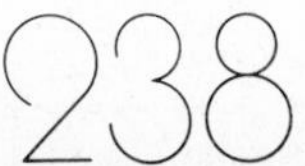

Table 13.1 SELECTED TERMINOLOGY OF THE GENITOURINARY SYSTEM

Bowman	glomerulus	seminal
bulbourethral	hilus	seminal vesicle
calyces	juxtaglomerular	seminiferous
calyx	labia	sperm
clitoris	menstrual	testis
convoluted	micturition	trigone
corpus luteum	nephron	ureter
ductus deferens	ovary	urethra
endometrium	oviduct	urinary
epididymis	ovulation	urination
Fallopian	ovum	uterus
follicle	papillary	vagina
fundus	penis	vas deferens
genitourinary	prostate	vulva
glans	pyramids	
glomerular	scrotum	

Glomerul/ar
(glō mer′ yə lər)

1040

______/___ "pertains to a little ball of yarn" in the same way that *alveolar* (frame 987) "pertains to tiny cavities."

proxim

juxta/glomerul/ar
(juks′ tə glō mer′ yə lər)

1041

Juxta, like ________ (frame 165), is a root for "near." We can build ______/______/___, a term "referring to (something) near the little ball of yarn," using this new root.

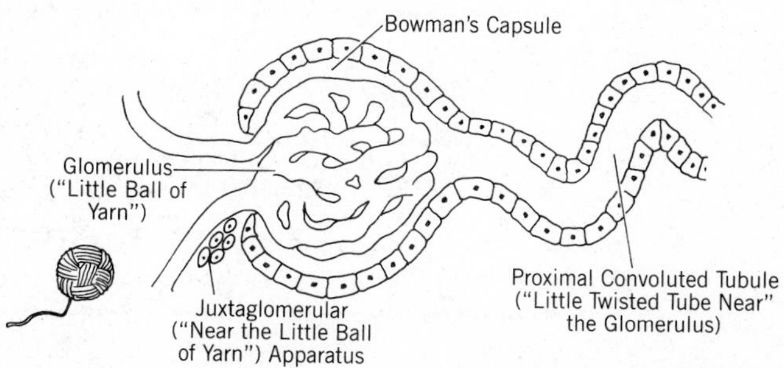

Figure 13.1. INITIAL PORTION OF* NEPHRON *("PRESENCE OF KIDNEY")

juxtaglomerular tubules	**1042** The ____________________ *apparatus* consists of a set of special receptor cells located "near" the "glomerulus" (Fig. 13.1). These cells monitor the Na^+ ion concentration within the kidney __________ ("small tubes," frame 233).
proximal distal	**1043** If something is *convoluted* (kon′ və lo͞ot′ əd) it is "twisted." You can probably guess that the __________ (proximal/distal) *convoluted tubule* is immediately adjacent to Bowman's capsule, whereas the ________ (proximal/distal) *convoluted tubule* lies farther down the line. Both of these tubes have a "twisted" appearance.
papill/ary (pap′ i ler ē)	**1044** Perhaps you remember that the root of *papilla* ("a small pimple," frames 384–385), like that of *epithelium* (frame 372), can mean "nipple." Using this first root plus the suffix of *salivary* (frame 997) we have ________/____ ("characterized by little nipples").
convoluted papillary	**1045** The *distal* ____________ ("twisted") *tubule* hooks into a *collecting duct*, which expands into a __________ ("little nipple") *duct*.
papilla	**1046** The *papillary duct* gets its name from the fact that groups of such ducts running alongside each other eventually taper into a __________ ("small nipple present") at the end (Fig. 13.2).
	1047 More like the flat-topped constructions of the Aztec Indians than the sharply pointed ____

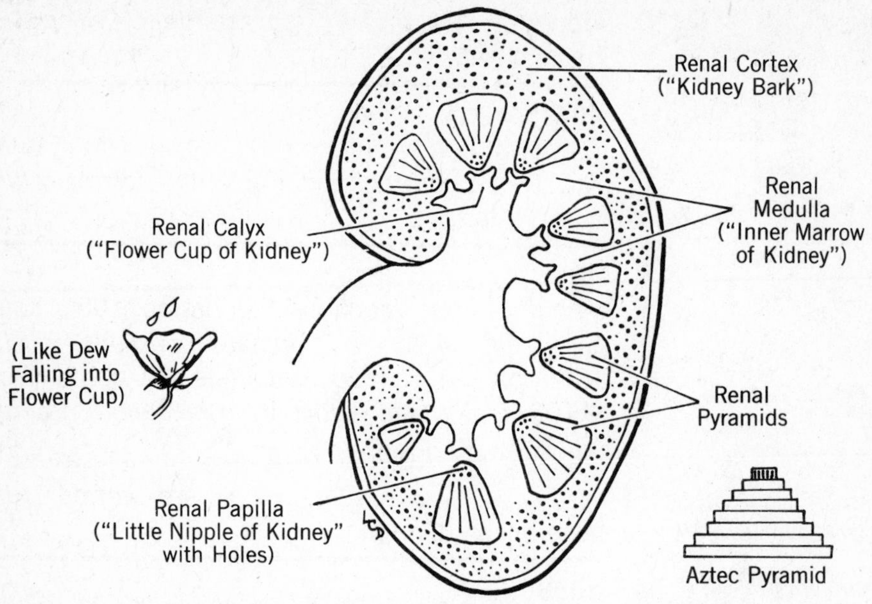

Figure 13.2. SAGITTAL SECTION OF KIDNEY

pyramids medulla	____________ of ancient Egypt, the collecting ducts and papillary ducts from different groups of nephrons form definite geometric structures within the *renal* ____________ ("presence of a middle or marrow," frame 833) (Fig. 13.2).
calyces (kā′ lisēz)	**1048** Words ending in *-yx* take plurals with *-yces*. Thus if *calyx* (kā′ liks) means "flower cup" then ____________ are "flower cups."
papilla calyx	**1049** The peak or ____________ ("little nipple") of each renal pyramid is full of holes like the top of a saltshaker. Urine flows through these holes into a waiting *renal* ________, like dew dripping into the "cup of a flower" (Fig. 13.2).
calyces	**1050** These small or *minor* ____________ ("cups") branch from *major* "cups" that extend like the tops of tulips growing from the

pelvis	kidney ________ ("presence of a bowl/basin," frame 59).
urine	**1051** *Urinat*, of course, means "________," just like *mictur, urethr*, and the entire term *ureter* (yoor′ e tar).
urinat/ion mictur/i/tion (mik tyə rish′ ən)	**1052** The first root mentioned in frame 1051 can take the suffix in *ventilation* (frame 978), whereas the second root uses the combining vowel *i* plus the suffix in *ossification* (frame 421). Thus both ________/____ and ________/__/____ are terms for "the act of urinating."
urethr/a (yoo rē′ thrə)	**1053** The third root mentioned in frame 1051 has the same "presence of" format as does *papill*. Hence ________/__ can be translated as "presence of urine."
urination micturition urethra	**1054** Before actual ________ or ________, "the act of" passing "urine" out of the body, the still unexcreted "urine" is "present" in the ________. This is simply a tube that begins in the bladder and carries the urine to its exit point from the body (Fig. 13.3).
ureter pelvis	**1055** The ________ (the entire term for "urine" in frame 1051) is the tube conducting urine from the *renal* ________ or "basin present" at a "trifle little" slit in the medial wall of the kidney (Fig. 13.3).
hil/us (hī′ ləs)	**1056** If *hil* means "small trifle" then ____/____ is a term for "presence of a small trifle," where

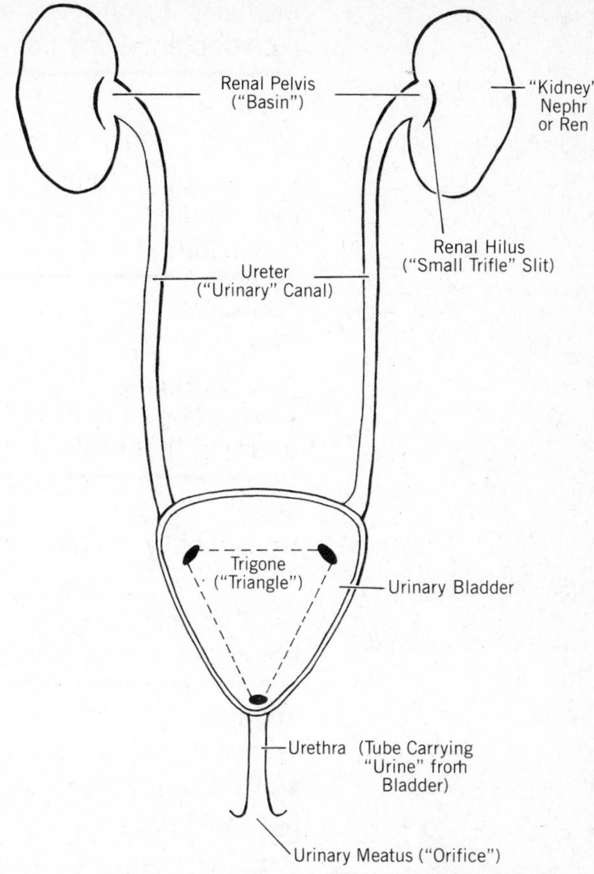

Figure 13.3. URINE PATHWAY

	the ending of *glomerulus* is the appropriate suffix.
Urin/ary papill/ary	**1057** ________/______ means "characterized by *urin*" just as __________/______ (frame 1044) is "characterized by *papill*."
hilus	**1058** Urine in the funnel-shaped *renal pelvis* passes out of the kidney through the *renal* __________, just a "small trifle" slit "present" in the medial kidney wall. The ureter then carries

urinary	the urine toward the waiting ______ ("characterized by urine") *bladder* (Fig. 13.3).
trigon/e (trī′ gōn)	**1059** If *trigon* means "triangle" then ______ /__ denotes "presence of a triangle," where the suffix of *leukocyte* (frame 916) is employed.
trigone	**1060** The ______ of the urinary bladder is the "triangular" region "present" between the three points made by the opening of the urethra and that of the two ureters (Fig. 13.3).
meatus	**1061** Urine finally leaves the body through a small ______ (frame 763) or "opening present" at the tip of the *penis* (pē′ nis) or just below the *clitoris* (klit′ ər is) in the female.
urinary genit/o/urin/ary (jen′ i tō yoor′ i ner ē)	**1062** The root and combining vowel *genit/o*, like the suffix of *agglutinogen* (frame 933), means "beget" or "produce." If ______ (frame 1057) is "characterized by urine" then ____/__/______/____ is "characterized by begetting and urinating."
test acorn	**1063** Consider the following roots: *pen* "tail" ______ "eggshell" (frame 814) or "witness" *didym* "eggshell" *clitor* "shut or closed in" *glans* "______" (same meaning as *gland*, frame 777)
	1064 All the roots in frame 1063 but the last take the "presence of" suffix in *pelvis* (frame 1050).

pen/is clitor/is	Thus ______/____ denotes "presence of a tail," while __________/____ describes the "presence of (something) shut or closed in."
glans penis	**1065** Urine leaves the male body through the meatus in the "acorn"-shaped ________ of the ________, an erectile structure "present" like a short "tail" on the anterior trunk (Fig. 13.4).
genitourinary	**1066** The penis is a ______________________ structure, "characterized by" its ability to both help "beget" new life and to excrete "urine."
Test/is	**1067** _______/____ is a single term denoting "presence of an eggshell or a witness." "Eggshell" comes from the appearance of each gland, while "witness" is oddly used because the gland bears "witness" or *test*ifies to a person's masculinity! After all, this structure does produce *sperm* ("seed")!
didym epi/didym/is (ep i did′ ə mis)	**1068** The prefix in *epiglottis* (frame 972) combines with _________, the root in frame 1063 for "eggshell" only, to result in ______/______ ____/____, "presence of (something) upon an eggshell."
epididymis sperm	**1069** The ________________ is a body consisting of convoluted tubules "present upon the eggshell"-like structure of the testis (Fig. 13.4). It stores _________ ("seed") between ejaculations.
	1070 *Scrot* means "bag" while *ov* like *ovi* (frame 407) is "egg." Each root can take the ending

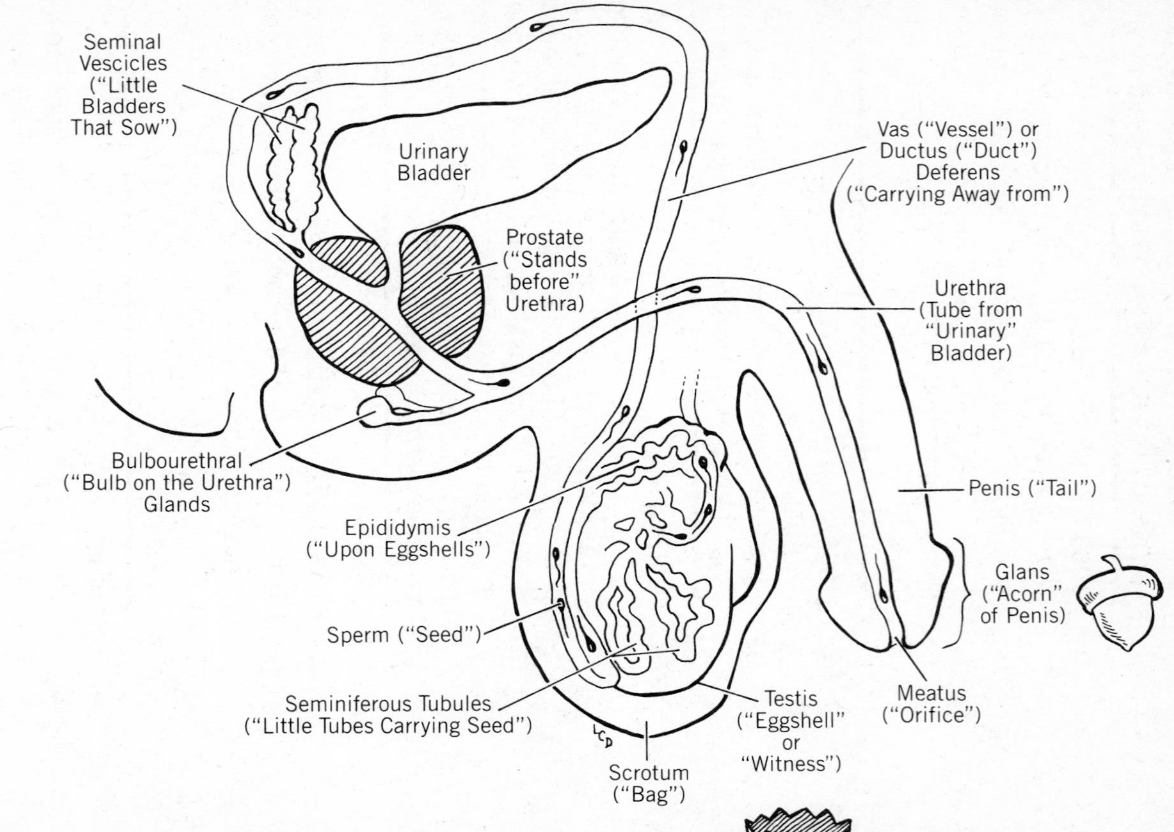

Figure 13.4. MALE SEXUAL APPARATUS (INTERIOR VIEW)

scrot/um (skrō′ təm)
ov/um (ō′ vəm)

in *omentum* (frame 1029). Thus ________/____ is "presence of a bag" while ____/____ is "presence of an egg."

---

testis
scrotum
ovum
ov/ary (ō′ vər ē)

1071
Each __________ resembles an oval white "eggshell present" within the __________, a hairy external "bag." The ________ is a tiny "egg present" within the female ____/______, an endocrine gland "characterized by eggs" just as *urinary* is "characterized by urine."

Semin/al (sem′ i nəl)
vesicle

1072
Semin means "seed" or "sow." ________/____ "pertains to sowing," where the suffix of *gastrointestinal* (frame 1014) is borrowed. Recall that a __________ (frame 240) is a "little bladder."

---

seminal vesicle

1073
A ____________________* is a "little bladder that sows," lying posterior to the urinary bladder and secreting a thick fluid into the urethra (Fig. 13.4). This fluid medium helps to "sow the seed" during ejaculation!

---

fer
De/fer/ens
semin/i/fer/ous

1074
Look at *seminiferous* (sem i nif′ ər əs) and *deferens* (def′ ər enz). Both have the root ______ ("to carry," frame 712) in common. The ending *-ens* means the same as the suffix in *efferent* (frame 714). ____/______/______ means "one that carries (something) away from," where the prefix is that in *deoxyribonucleic* (frames 333–335). And ________/____/______/______ "pertains to the carrying of seed," just as *venous* (frame 868) "pertains to poison."

---

seminiferous

1075
The ______________ *tubules* are "little tubes that carry sperm" out of each tes-

Vas deferens ductus deferens	tis into the *epididymis*. ______________ ______* (Vas deferens/Ductus deferens) is the phrase used for "vessel carrying (sperm) away from," while ______________ __________* (vas deferens/ductus deferens) is the phrase indicating a "duct carrying (sperm) away from." Both phrases describe the same tube carying sperm away from the epididymis and into the urethra (Fig. 13.4).
pro/stat/e (pros′ tāt)	**1076** If *stat* is a root for "stand" then _____/ ________/__ indicates the "presence of (something) standing in front or before." Both the prefix and the last letter of this term are found in *prophase* (frame 344).
bulb/o/urethr/al	**1077** Referring back to Figure 13.4, you can see that ________/__/____________/____ literally "pertains to a bulb on the urethra."
prostate bulbourethral	**1078** The _______________ *gland* "stands before" the urethra at the inferior neck of the bladder. And the two ______________ *glands* form twin "bulbs" on the same channel. All these glands add fluid to the sperm.
vagin/a (və jī′ nə)	**1079** During sexual intercourse, the penis is inserted into the __________/__, an opening "present" in the female reproductive system. For help in filling the blank of the preceding sentence, choose the most appropriate root below: *labi* "lip" *vulv* "wrapper" *vagin* "sheath" All of these roots take the "presence of" suffix in *urethra* (frame 1053).

vulva vagina labia (lā′ bē ə) clitoris	**1080** The ________ is the "wrapper present" around the ________, a slick "sheath" that receives the blunt tool of the penis. This female genital "wrapper" includes the "presence of lips" or ________, which at least partially "shut or close in" around the ________ (frame 1064).
body lute	**1081** Look at these roots for internal female reproductive structures: *uter* "womb" *corp* "________" (same meaning as for *somat*, frame 783) fund "base/bottom" of an organ ________ "yellow" (frame 740) All the roots in this frame take the "presence of" ending in *hilus* (frame 1056), except for the last root, which takes the suffix of *ovum*.
uter/us (yōō′ tər əs)	**1082** The ________/____ is the "womb present" within the abdominal cavity of the female. It looks much like an inverted 3-inch pear.
uterus sperm vagina	**1083** A "womb" is generally considered a structure that holds, envelopes, or generates something. Just as the soft fleshy "womb" of a ripe pear envelopes hidden fruit seeds, the ________ ("womb present") in a human female envelopes ________ ("seeds") ejaculated into the ________ ("a sheath") (Fig. 13.5).
fund/us (fun′ dəs)	**1084** The ________/____ forms the broad "base" or "bottom present" on the hollow pear of the uterus. But the *cervix* (sûr′ viks) forms the narrow "neck" of the pear just as the ________

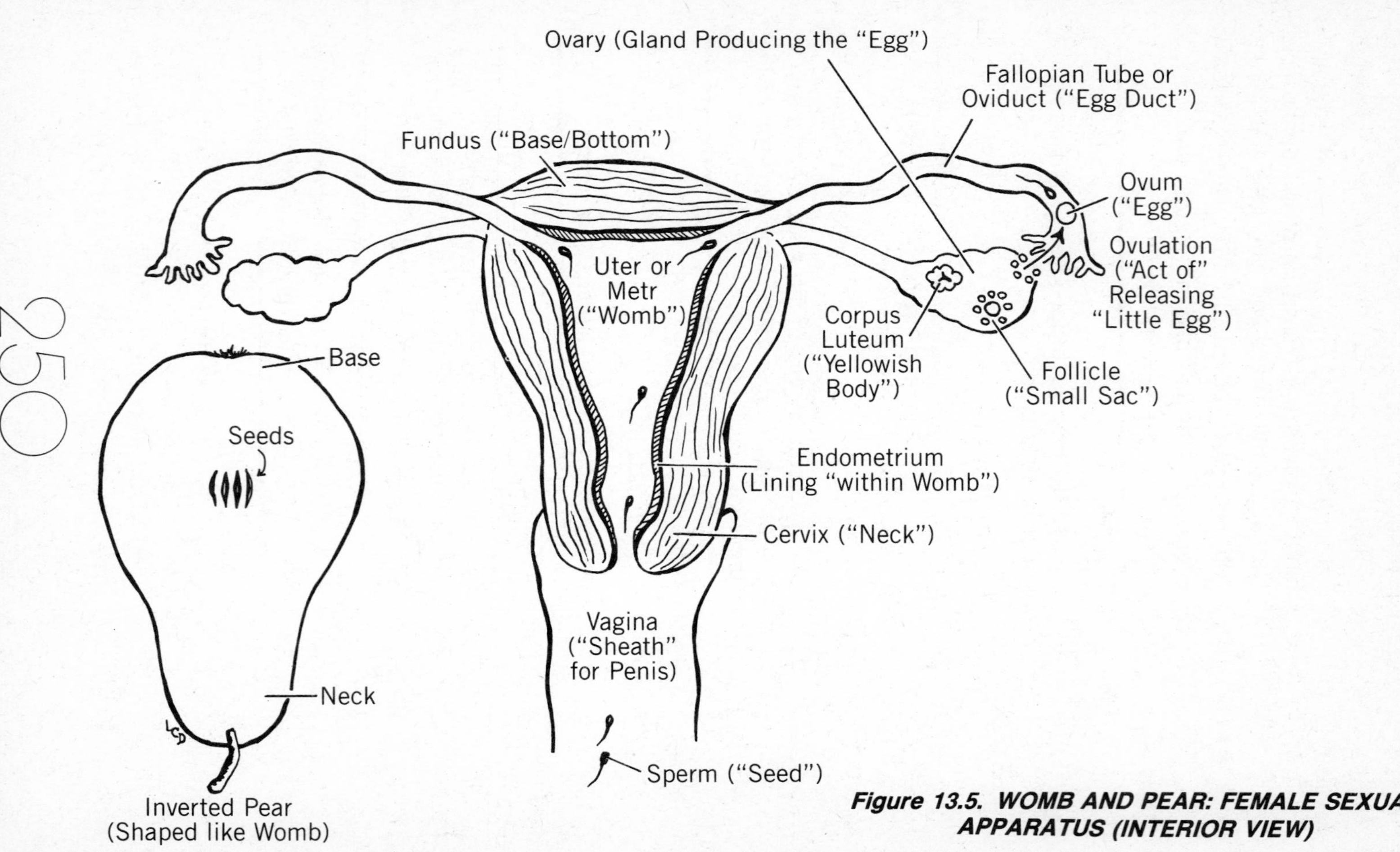

Figure 13.5. WOMB AND PEAR: FEMALE SEXUAL APPARATUS (INTERIOR VIEW)

cervical	________ (frame 468) *vertebrae* form the "neck" under the human head (Fig. 13.5).
corpus luteum (kôr′ pəs lo͞ot′ ē əm)	**1085** From frame 1081 you can build ________ ________,* which translates as "presence of a yellow body."
globul ovum	**1086** If *ov* (frame 1070) is a root for "egg" then *ovulat* is a root for "little egg," since it includes *ul* as in ________ ("little globe," frame 940). In actual practice these two roots mean the same, since the ________ ("egg presence") is quite tiny and microscopic!
ovulat/ion (ov yo͞o lā′ shən)	**1087** For exact translation, however, we would say that ________/________ is "the act of (releasing) a little egg" just as *urinat/ion* (frame 1052) is "the act of (releasing) urine."
follic/le (fol′ i kəl)	**1088** If *follic* means "sac" then ________/ ________ must mean "little sac," in the same manner that *vesicle* (frame 240) is a "little bladder."
follicle ovulation ovum corpus luteum	**1089** Each month a mature ________ (spherical mass of cells resembling a "little sac" within the ovary) undergoes ________ ________ (the "process of" releasing a "little egg"). After the ________ ("egg") has been released, the remnant of the "little sac" still in the ovary transforms into a ________ ________* ("yellowish body" that secretes hormones) (Fig. 13.5).
ovum sperm	**1090** Fertilization of the ________ ("egg") by a ________ ("seed") generally occurs in the

Answers	Frames
ov/i/duct (ō′ vi dukt)	upper third of the ____/__/______ ("egg duct;" use the combining vowel *i*).
Fallopi/an (fə lō′ pē ən) Havers/i/an	**1091** This *oviduct* is often called the ______/____ *tube* after its discoverer, the sixteen-century Italian anatomist, Gabriel *Fallopius* (fa lō′ pē əs). This is similar to ______/__/____ ("referring to *Havers*," frame 443).
menstru/al (men′ stroo əl)	**1092** If *menstru* means "month" then ______/____ is a term for "monthly," where the adjectival suffix is the same as that in *seminal*.
progesterone menstrual	**1093** The glandular *corpus luteum* is an important source of ____________ ("before-bearing steroid," frames 815–816) in the latter part of the female ____________ ("monthly") *cycle*.
uter endo/metr/i/um (en dō mē′ trē əm) endo/neur/i/um	**1094** *Metr*, like ________, is a root for "womb." We use the first root to name the various layers of the womb's wall. For example, we have the ______/______/__/____ or "presence within womb" just as we had the ______/______/__/____ ("presence within nerve," frame 694).
endometrium	**1095** If fertilization of the ovum by a sperm has occurred, the resultant "seed of life" is planted in the ____________ ("inner uterine" lining) and the cycle of human life begins anew.

Now do the Self-Test for Unit 13 (page 282 in the Appendix).

UNIT 14
TERMS OF HUMAN DEVELOPMENT

Answers	Frame
zygot/e (zī′ gōt) neo/nat/e (nē′ ō nāt)	**1096** *Neo* means "new." Both *zygot* ("yoked") and *nat* ("birth/born") take the "presence of" ending in *prostate* (frame 1076). Thus ________ /__ indicates the "presence of" two or more structures "yoked" together, while ______/ ______/__ describes the "presence of a newborn."
sperm ovum zygote mitosis neonate	**1097** Both __________ ("seed," frame 1067) and ________ ("egg," frame 1070) are fused and "yoked" to form a single ____________ "present" after fertilization. Successive ________ ______ ("condition of threads," frame 340) of this original body cell eventually produces a ______________ ("newborn present") in the world!
gastr blast	**1098** Recall from frame 1014 that __________ is a root for "stomach." *Mor* means "mulberry," and you should already know that the __________ in *fibroblast* (frame 355) means "sprout."
	1099 Each of the roots in frame 1098 becomes "little" like *ov* did in *ovul* (frame 1086). And each of these "little" roots is "present" like *vulva*

Table 14.1 BASIC TERMS OF HUMAN DEVELOPMENT

allantois	embryo	morula
amnion	endoderm	neonate
blastocyst	fetal	placenta
blastula	fetus	zygote
chorionic villi	gastrula	
ectoderm	mesoderm	

morul/a (môr′ yə lə)

(frames 1079–1080). Consequently, we have the ________/__, a solid mass of developing cells that looks much like a "little mulberry present" in the *endometrium* (Fig. 14.1).

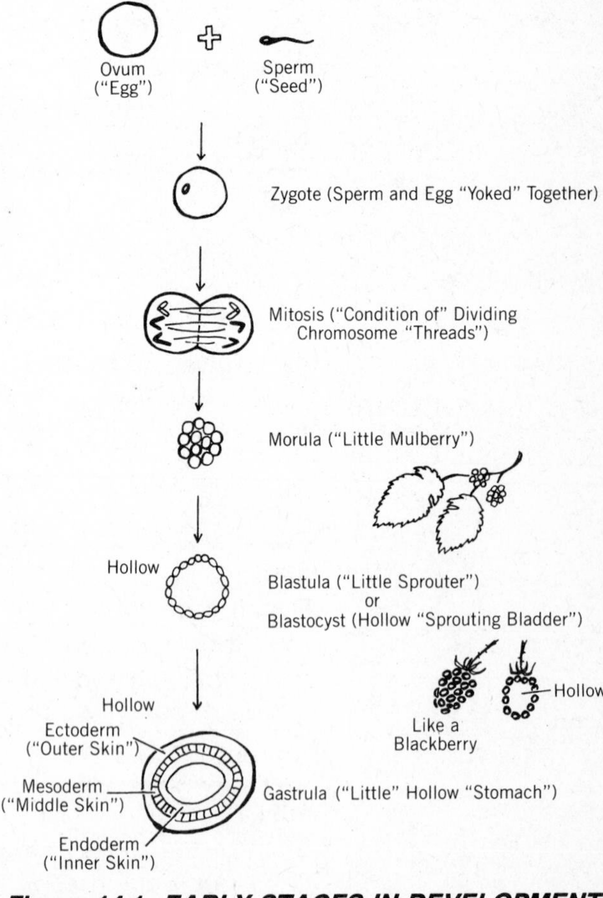

Figure 14.1. EARLY STAGES IN DEVELOPMENT

Answers	Frame
blastul/a (blas′ tyə lə) gastrul/a (gas′ trə lə)	**1100** And we have the ____________/__ or "little sprouter present" later as a hollow sphere of dividing cells. Finally the ____________/__ is the "little stomach present" with three different layers in its wall.
morula blastula	**1101** As you can see from Figure 14.1, if the ____________ looks like a solid "little mulberry" then the ____________ resembles a hollow "little" blackberry or raspberry "sprouted" in the summer garden!
bladder blast/o/cyst (blas′ tō sist)	**1102** *Cyst*, like *vesic* (frame 239), is a root for "____________." Therefore __________/__/________ or "sprouting bladder" (using connecting *o*) is an alternate name for *blastula*.
blastocyst gastrula	**1103** The ____________ is like a miniature "bladder" that "sprouts" three different layers, becoming a ____________ ("little stomach") in the process.
germinativum	**1104** The three primary *germ* layers of the gastrula, like the *stratum* ____________ of the *epidermis* (frames 399–400), give rise to many other cell types via the process of mitosis.
derm	**1105** Each *germ* layer of the gastrula is described as a different kind of ________ (root for "skin" in *epidermis*).
endo/derm (en′ dō dûrm) endo/cardi/um	**1106** The ________/________ is the "inner skin" of the gastrula just as the ________/________/____ (frame 876) is the "inner heart" lining.

mes/o/derm
(mez′ ō dûrm)

mes/encephal/on

1107
The ______/__/______ is the "middle skin" in a manner like the ______/______/____ (frame 625) is the "middle brain."

ecto-

1108
You learned way back in frame 40 that ________, the prefix in *ectopelvic*, means "outside of."

ecto/derm
(ek′ tō dûrm)

1109
Consequently, the ______/______ must refer to the "outer skin" of the developing *embryo* ("in swelling") (Fig. 14.1).

embryo (em′ brē ō)

zygote

1110
This __________ represents all cells "in" the act of "swelling" their numbers by active division, from the __________ ("yoked" cells) up through the end of the second month of human development.

ectoderm

1111
The ____________ (endoderm/mesoderm/ectoderm) "swells" and differentiates to form much of the nervous system and other structures in intimate contact with the "external" environment.

mesoderm

1112
The ____________ (endoderm/mesoderm/ectoderm) "swells" to form bones, muscle, and other structures located in the "middle" of the body.

endoderm

1113
And the ____________ (endoderm/mesoderm/ectoderm) "swells" to form the "inner" lining of the digestive tract and similar systems.

1114
The developing embryo is associated with

chor	three protective membranes whose roots are as follows: *amni* "lamb" ________ (frame 750) "membrane" *allant* "sausage"
Amni/on (am′ nē on) Chor/i/on (kō′ rē on)	**1115** ________/____ represents "presence of a lamb," where the suffix is that in *nephron* (frame 1037). ________/__/____ ("presence of a membrane") is formed in like manner, except for the addition of a connecting *i* between root and suffix.
Allant/ois (ə lan′ tō is)	**1116** ____________/______ ("resembling a sausage") has a suffix identical to that in *choroid* (frame 750) except that the terminal *-d* is replaced by *-s*.
amnion	**1117** No doubt the early Greeks and Romans, being nomadic peoples with large wandering herds of goats and sheep, must have noticed the ____________, an inner sac filled with fluid "present" around the undelivered "lamb" (Fig. 14.2).
allantois chorion	**1118** And some observer thought that the ____ ____________, a narrow tubelike structure, "resembled a sausage"! This thin "sausage" extends from the yolk sac of the embryo into the stalk that connects it to the inner surface of the ____________ ("a membrane") (Fig. 14.2).
chorion	**1119** The ____________ is the outermost "membrane present" around the amnion, allantois, and embryo.

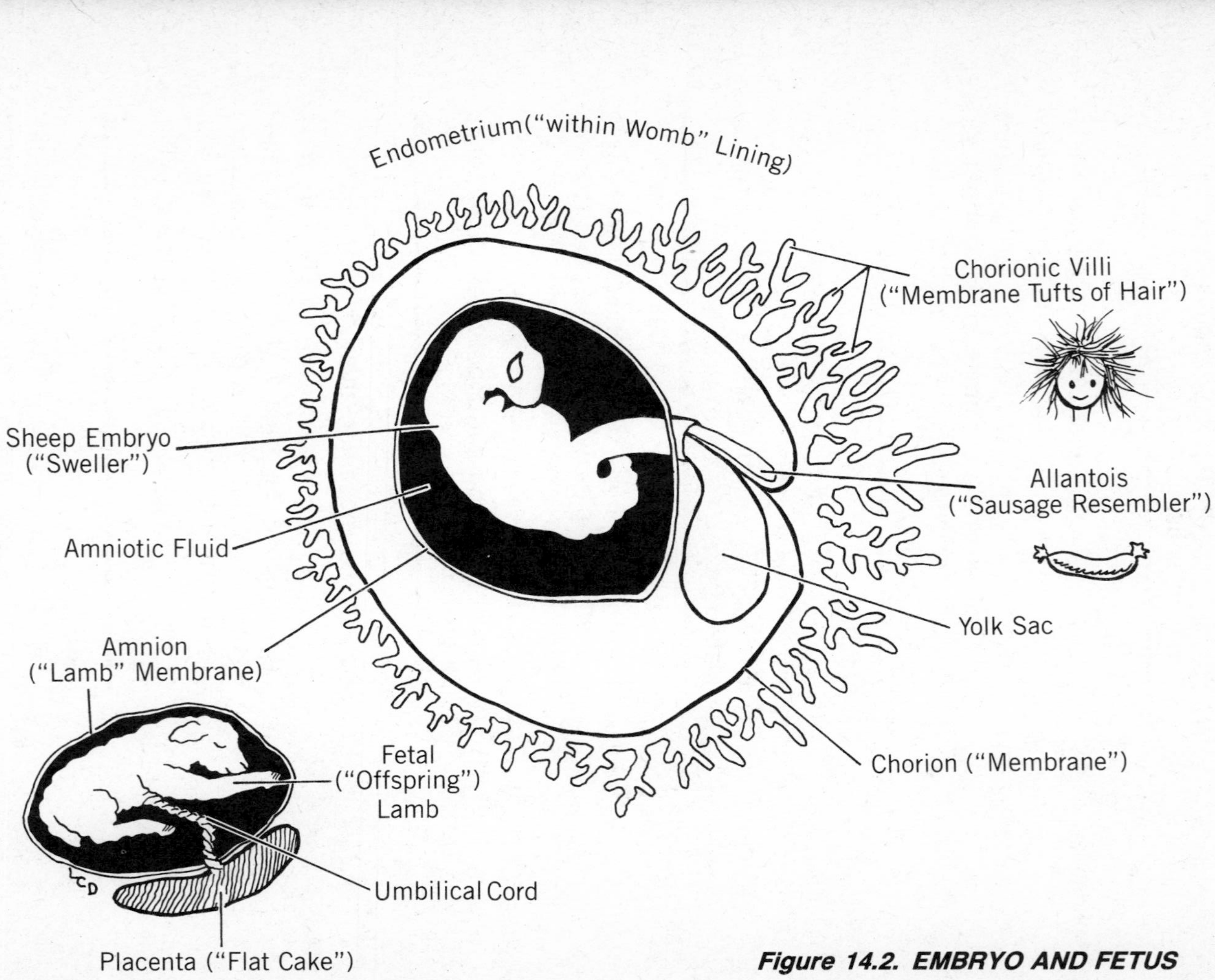

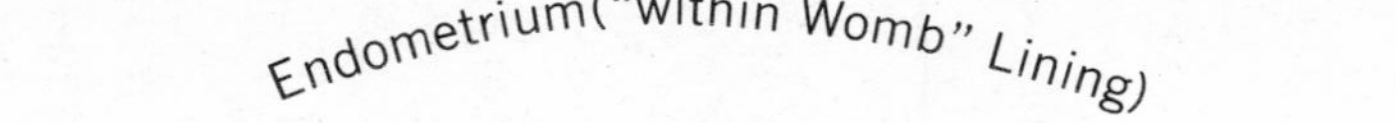

Figure 14.2. ***EMBRYO AND FETUS***

villi

1120
You know that __________ (frame 1032) are literally "tufts of hair" if you have already studied the digestive system.

---

chorionic villi

endometrium

1121
Chorion can take the suffix in *splenic* (frame 1019). Thus the ________________________ ______* "refer to membrane tufts of hair" that extend like slender fingers into the __________ ____________ ("inner" lining of the "womb," frame 1095) (Fig. 14.2).

---

fet/us (fē′ təs)

fet/al

umbilicus

umbilical

1122
If *fet* is a root for "offspring" then ______/____ denotes "presence of an offspring" and ______/____ "pertains to an offspring." These two terms bear the same relationship to each other as do ________________ ("presence of a pit," frame 120) and ____________ ______ ("pertaining to a pit," frame 121).

---

fetus

embryo

1123
The developing human being "present" within the uterus is called a __________ ("offspring") rather than an ____________ ("sweller") from the beginning of the third month after fertilization to the actual time of birth.

---

placent/a (plə sen′ tə)

1124
If *placent* means "flat cake" then ______ ________/__ denotes "presence of a flat cake" just as *blastula* (frame 1100) denotes "presence of a little sprouter."

---

allantois

placenta

umbilical

1125
The "sausage-like" ________________ contributes to the development of both the ________________ ("a flat cake") and the ________________ ("referring to pit/navel")

fetal	*cord*. These structures are crucial for ______ ("offspring") survival!
chorionic villi placenta	**1126** Those ______________________* ("hair tufts" of the outer fetal "membrane") in contact with the endometrium become part of the ______________, a heavy oval organ shaped like "a flat cake" (Fig. 14.2). This temporary organ acts in the transfer of wastes and nutrients between the maternal and fetal bloodstreams.
umbilical placenta	**1127** The ______________ ("navel") *cord* connects the circulation in the "midriff" of the fetus to the ______________ (intrauterine "pancake") of its mother, through which it derives nourishment.
fetus vagina	**1128** The ________ or immature child soon to be born as an "offspring" passes out through the __________ (frame 1079), a "sheath present" in its mother.
neonate	**1129** Right after birth the fetus becomes a ______________ (frame 1096) or "newborn present" for the very first time in the external world!
	1130 You have been learning an extensive system of anatomical and physiological terminology that has slowly evolved over the centuries to describe the body. This systematic learning process in many ways imitates the gradual step-by-step unfolding of potential in the amazing human being from the point of its first conception.

Now do the Self-Test for Unit 14 (page 283 in the Appendix).

APPENDIX UNIT SELF-TESTS

The following exercises test for word parts and plurals as they appear for the *first time* within the units. You may want to work from the word part itself or from its English equivalent. Cover either the right-hand or the left-hand side of each page with a piece of paper. Go back and rework previous self-tests often. You will gradually build a powerful vocabulary of body nomenclature.

For review of entire terms and related concepts, simply re-do the appropriate frames in the units themselves.

UNIT 1: SELF-TEST OF WORD PARTS

PREFIXES	MEANING	
ana-	__________	"up; toward; apart"
epi-	__________	"upon"
hypo-	__________	"below"
trans-	__________	"across"

ROOTS	MEANING	
bucc	__________	"cheek"
or	__________	"mouth"
gastr	__________	"stomach"
chondr	__________	"cartilage"
viscer	__________	"internal organs"
pariet	__________	"wall"
pelv	__________	"bowl"
tom	__________	"cut"

ROOTS	MEANING	
abdomin	______________	"trunk midsection"
umbilic	______________	"pit"
coron	______________	"crown"
dors	______________	"back"
anter	______________	"front"
poster	______________	"behind; rear"
ventr	______________	"belly"
later	______________	"side"
medi	______________	"middle" (contains *d*)
mes	______________	"middle" (contains *s*)
crani	______________	"skull"
cephal	______________	"head"
vertebr	______________	"jointed backbone"
ili	______________	"flank"
vers	______________	"turn"
sutur	______________	"seam"
infer	______________	"below"
super	______________	"above"
thorac	______________	"chest"
sagitt	______________	"arrow"
caud	______________	"tail"
lumb	______________	"loins"
homeo	______________	"sameness"
physi	______________	"nature"
log	______________	"study"
proxim	______________	"near"
dist	______________	"distant"

ROOTS	MEANING	
intern	______________	"inside of"
extern	______________	"outside of"

SUFFIXES	MEANING	
-y	______________	"action, process, or condition of"
-al	______________	"pertaining to" (2 letters; ends with *l*)
-ical	______________	"pertaining to" (ends with *al*)
-ar	______________	"pertaining to" (ends with *r*)
-ic	______________	"pertaining to" (2 letters; starts with *i*)
-ac	______________	"pertaining to" (ends with *c*)
-stasis	______________	"control of"
-ion	______________	"the act or process of"
-ology	______________	"the study of"
-or	______________	"one which; one who"
-us	______________	"presence of" (ends with *s*)
-um	______________	"presence of" (ends with *m*)
-e	______________	"presence of" (1 letter)

UNIT 2: SELF-TEST OF WORD PARTS

PREFIXES	MEANING	
mono-	______________	"single"
di-	______________	"double; two"

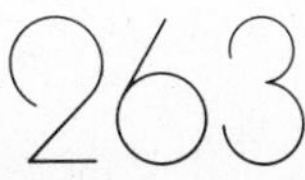

PREFIXES	MEANING	
tri-	____________	"three"
iso-	____________	"same; equal"
hyper-	____________	"above normal; excessive"
semi-	____________	"partially"
de-	____________	"away from"
poly-	____________	"many"
extra-	____________	"outside of"
intra-	____________	"within; inside of"
endo-	____________	"within; inside of" (starts with *e*)
meta-	____________	"after"
pro-	____________	"before; first"
telo-	____________	"end"
inter-	____________	"between"
a-	____________	"not; without" (1 letter)
in-	____________	"not"

ROOTS	MEANING	
lyt	____________	"breakdown" (ends with *t*)
lys	____________	"breakdown" (ends with *s*)
molec	____________	"mass"
mei	____________	"lessening"
mit	____________	"thread"
electr	____________	"electricity"
crist	____________	"comb; crest"
som	____________	"body"
protein	____________	"first"

ROOTS	MEANING	
oxy	________	"oxygen"
centr	________	"central"
cyt	________	"cell"
plasm	________	"matter"
cellul	________	"small chamber"
reticul	________	"little network"
nucle	________	"kernel"
nucleol	________	"little kernel"
chrom	________	"colored"
micr	________	"tiny"
rib	________	"a 5-carbon sugar" (ribose)
vesic	________	"bladder"
vac	________	"empty space"
bio	________	"life"
ton	________	"strength"
osm	________	"thrusting"
diffus	________	"spreading out; scattering"
phag	________	"eat"
pin	________	"drink"
tub	________	"tube"
chem	________	"chemical"
phosph	________	"phosphorus"
solv	________	"dissolve" (ends with *v*)
solut	________	"dissolve" (ends with *t*)
lip	________	"fat"
ion	________	"going; carrying"

ROOTS	MEANING	
carb	____________	"carbon"
hydr	____________	"water"
sacchar	____________	"sugar"
glyc	____________	"sweetness"
genet	____________	"produce" (ends with *t*)
gen	____________	"produce"

SUFFIXES	MEANING	
-ent	____________	"one that"
-gen	____________	"produce"
-ate	____________	"something that"
-id	____________	"belonging to a group"
-ide	____________	"compound with 2 different parts"
-osis	____________	"condition of"
-ase	____________	"splitter"
-mere	____________	"segment"
-ule	____________	"tiny" (starts with *u*)
-ole	____________	"tiny" (starts with *o*)
-le	____________	"tiny" (starts with *l*)
-elle	____________	"tiny; miniature"
-able	____________	"able"
-on	____________	"presence of" (ends with *n*)

SINGULAR		PLURAL
mitochondrion	____________	mitochondria
crista	____________	cristae

UNIT 3: SELF-TEST OF WORD PARTS

PREFIXES	MEANING	
syn	______________	"together"
sub	______________	"below; beneath; under"

ROOTS	MEANING	
gross	______________	"large" (starts with *g*)
macr	______________	"large" (starts with *m*)
scop	______________	"examine"
hist	______________	"web; tissue"
areol	______________	"little area"
blast	______________	"sprout; forms"
germinativ	______________	"sprout" (starts with *g*)
colla	______________	"glue"
elast	______________	"stretch"
adipos	______________	"fat"
fasci	______________	"band; sheet"
fibr	______________	"fiber"
cub	______________	"cube"
theli	______________	"nipple"
squam	______________	"scale"
gland	______________	"acorn"
glandul	______________	"little acorn"
seb	______________	"grease"
sebac	______________	"grease" (ends with *c*)
papill	______________	"small pimple"
ser	______________	"whey"

ROOTS	MEANING	
muc	______________	"slime"
strat	______________	"layer; bedcover"
ovi	______________	"egg"
bas	______________	"base; bottom"
corne	______________	"horny"
lucid	______________	"clear"
spinos	______________	"spine; thorn"
granulos	______________	"little grain"
derm	______________	"skin" (ends with *m*)
cori	______________	"skin" (ends with *i*)
cutan	______________	"skin" (ends with *n*)
cutic	______________	"skin" (ends with *c*)
cut	______________	"skin" (ends with *t*)

SUFFIXES	MEANING	
-is	______________	"presence of"
-a	______________	"presence of" (1 letter)
-ous	______________	"pertaining to"
-oid	______________	"resembling"

SINGULAR		PLURAL
stratum	______________	strata

UNIT 4: SELF-TEST OF WORD PARTS

PREFIXES	MEANING	
dia-	______________	"through"
peri-	______________	"around"

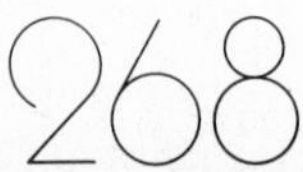

ROOTS	MEANING	
glen	________	"socket"
skelet	________	"dried body"
capit	________	"head"
capitul	________	"little head"
trochle	________	"pulley"
cervic	________	"neck"
ax	________	"axle; axis"
appendicul	________	"little attachment"
galli	________	"rooster"
membran	________	"membrane"
cartilagin	________	"cartilage"
fic	________	"make"
arthr	________	"joint"
articul	________	"little joint"
burs	________	"leather sack; purse"
odont	________	"tooth" (ends with *t*)
dens	________	"tooth" (ends with *s*)
styl	________	"stake; pole; pillar"
mast	________	"breast"
corac	________	"crow; raven"
xiph	________	"sword" (contains *i*)
xyph	________	"sword" (contains *y*)
ethm	________	"sieve" (starts with *e*)
cribr	________	"sieve" (starts with *c*)
pis	________	"pea"
scapul	________	"shoulder blade"
clast	________	"break"

ROOTS	MEANING	
lacun	______	"small lake"
lamell	______	"little plate"
medull	______	"middle"
hyal	______	"glassy"
sell	______	"saddle"
turcic	______	"Turkey"
canalicul	______	"little canal"
phys	______	"growth"
oste	______	"bone" (contains one *s*)
osse	______	"bone" (contains *ss* and ends with *e*)
ossi	______	"bone" (contains *ss* and ends with *i*)
stern	______	"chest"
tempor	______	"temple"
pteryg	______	"wing"
hy	______	"the letter U"
foss	______	"trench; ditch; depression"
humer	______	"shoulder"
condyl	______	"knuckle"
acromi	______	"shoulder tip"
sphen	______	"wedge"

SUFFIXES	MEANING	
-form	______	"form; like"
-tion	______	"the act or process of"
-an	______	"pertaining to" (ends with *n*)

SUFFIXES	MEANING	
-ary	________	"pertaining to" (ends with *y*)
-ine	________	"pertaining to" (ends with *e*)

SINGULAR		PLURAL
lacuna	________	lacunae
canaliculus	________	canaliculi
lamella	________	lamellae

UNIT 5: SELF-TEST OF WORD PARTS

PREFIXES	MEANING	
ab-	________	"away from"
ad-	________	"toward"
bi-	________	"two"
quadri-	________	"four"

ROOTS	MEANING	
my	________	"muscle"
myos	________	"muscle" (contains *yo*)
mys	________	"mouse; muscle" (contains *ys*)
musc	________	"mouse; muscle" (ends with *c*)
muscul	________	"little mouse" (muscle)
sarc	________	"flesh" (muscle)
neur	________	"nerve"

ROOTS	MEANING	
ligament	________	"band; bandage"
fascic	________	"band; sheet"
tibi	________	"shin bone"
cost	________	"rib"
brachi	________	"arm"
pector	________	"breast; chest"
glute	________	"buttock"
gastrocnemi	________	"calf"
sole	________	"sandal; sole of foot"
tend	________	"stretcher"
extens	________	"stretching out; straightening out"
flex	________	"bending"
clavic	________	"key" (ends with *c*)
cleid	________	"key" (ends with *d*)
masset	________	"chew"
lemm	________	"husk"
metr	________	"length"
duct	________	"movement"
act	________	"motion"
rect	________	"vertical"
obliqu	________	"slanted"
buccinat	________	"trumpet"
fus	________	"spindle"
orbicul	________	"little orbit"
trapez	________	"table"
femor	________	"thigh"

SUFFIXES	MEANING	
-er	________	"a thing that"
-il	________	"tiny; little; small"
-in	________	"a neutral substance"
-alis	________	"pertaining to"

UNIT 6: SELF-TEST OF WORD PARTS

PREFIXES	MEANING	
af-	________	"toward"
ef-	________	"out of; away from"
auto-	________	"self"
en-	________	"inside of; within"
met-	________	"after"
tel-	________	"end"
para-	________	"beside"

ROOTS	MEANING	
synaps	________	"coming together" (ends with *s*)
synapt	________	"coming together" (ends with *t*)
gli	________	"glue"
gangli	________	"knot"
cortic	________	"cortex"
dendrit	________	"tree"
mid	________	"middle"
cerebr	________	"brain" (cerebrum)
cerebell	________	"little brain"

ROOTS	MEANING	
spin	________	"spinal cord"
myel	________	"spinal cord; marrow"
gyr	________	"circle; ring"
sulc	________	"furrow; ditch; wrinkle"
mening	________	"membrane"
pia	________	"tender; gentle"
dura	________	"hard; tough"
arachn	________	"spider's web"
mater	________	"mother"
thalam	________	"bedroom; inner chamber"
optic	________	"eye" (ends with *c*)
ocul	________	"eye" (ends with *l*)
chiasm	________	"Greek *X* or *chi*"
pituit	________	"mucus; phlegm"
hypophys	________	"undergrowth"
mammill	________	"little breast; nipple"
pedunc	________	"foot"
nerv	________	"nerve"
gloss	________	"tongue"
fer	________	"carry"
nom	________	"regulating"
ventric	________	"belly"
oblongat	________	"oblong"
somat	________	"body" (starts with *s*)
corpor	________	"body" (starts with *c*)
gemin	________	"twin"
collicul	________	"little hill"

ROOTS	MEANING	
audit	________	"hear" (ends with *it*)
acoust	________	"hear" (ends with *st*)
vag	________	"wander"
olfact	________	"smell"
pharynge	________	"throat"
cochle	________	"snail shell"
vestibul	________	"little entrance room"

SUFFIXES	MEANING	
-ary	________	"characterized by" (starts with *a*)
-ory	________	"characterized by"

SINGULAR		PLURAL
sulcus	________	sulci
gyrus	________	gyri
ganglion	________	ganglia
colliculus	________	colliculi

UNIT 7: SELF-TEST OF WORD PARTS

ROOTS	MEANING	
ossic	________	"bone"
labyrinth	________	"maze"
palpebr	________	"winker" (eyelid)
conjunctiv	________	"bind together"
aque	________	"water"
vitre	________	"glassy"
chor	________	"membrane"

ROOTS	MEANING	
tympan	______________	"drum"
auric	______________	"ear"
meat	______________	"opening; passage"
pup	______________	"girl; doll"
ir	______________	"rainbow"
fove	______________	"pit"
pinn	______________	"wing"
scler	______________	"hard"
cili	______________	"hair; eyelash"
retin	______________	"net"
macul	______________	"spot"
lute	______________	"yellow"
utric	______________	"skin bag"
sacc	______________	"sac"
malle	______________	"mallet; hammer"
inc	______________	"anvil"

UNIT 8: SELF-TEST OF WORD PARTS

PREFIXES	MEANING	
pan-	______________	"all"
anti-	______________	"against"
exo-	______________	"external; outside of"

ROOTS	MEANING	
insul	______________	"little island"
crin	______________	"secretion"

ROOTS	MEANING	
toc	______	"birth"
gest	______	"beget"
diuret	______	"urine through"
hormon	______	"arousal; setting into motion"
estr	______	"mad desire"
lact	______	"milk"
oxy	______	"swift; oxygen"
test	______	"eggshell"
troph	______	"nourish; feed"
trop	______	"turn; change"
cortis	______	"cortex"
gluc	______	"sweet" (ends with *c*)
glucag	______	"sweet" (ends with *g*)
ald	______	"aldehyde"
ren	______	"kidney" (starts with *r*)
nephr	______	"kidney" (starts with *n*)
thyr	______	"shield"
thyrox	______	"shield" (ends with *x*)
thym	______	"sweetbread"

SUFFIXES	MEANING	
-ose	______	"a type of sugar or other carbohydrate"
-ol	______	"alcohol; related to alcohol"
-ine (chemistry)	______	"a basic substance"
-sterone	______	"steroid"

UNIT 9: SELF-TEST OF WORD PARTS

ROOTS	MEANING	
tunic	__________	"coat; sheath"
lun	__________	"moon"
mitr	__________	"a Bishop's mitre"
dilat	__________	"widen"
constrict	__________	"narrow"
cav	__________	"cave"
sin	__________	"curve; bay"
vas	__________	"vessel"
cardi	__________	"heart"
aort	__________	"lifting up"
arter	__________	"windpipe"
pulmon	__________	"lung"
lumen	__________	"light space"
ven	__________	"vein; poison"
capill	__________	"hair"
atri	__________	"room; entrance room"
systol	__________	"contraction"
diastol	__________	"relaxation"
cuspid	__________	"point; tooth"
ventricul	__________	"little belly"

SINGULAR		PLURAL
atrium	__________	atria
artery	__________	arteries

UNIT 10: SELF-TEST OF WORD PARTS

ROOTS	MEANING	
vascul	____________	"vessel" ("little vessel")
erythr	____________	"red"
leuk	____________	"white"
album	____________	"egg white"
lymph	____________	"clear spring water"
lymphat	____________	"clear spring water" (ends with *t*)
thromb	____________	"clot"
glob	____________	"globe"
globul	____________	"little globe"
immun	____________	"exempt"
eosin	____________	"dawn"
phil	____________	"love"
agglutin	____________	"glue"
hem	____________	"blood"
hemat	____________	"blood" (ends with *t*)

SUFFIXES	MEANING	
-ity	____________	"condition of being"
-poiesis	____________	"formation of"

UNIT 11: SELF-TEST OF WORD PARTS

PREFIXES	MEANING	
re-	____________	"back; again"
ex-	____________	"out"
in-	____________	"in"

ROOTS	MEANING	
trache	____________	"rough artery; windpipe"
bronch	____________	"windpipe"
laryng	____________	"upper windpipe" (ends with *g*)
larynge	____________	"upper windpipe" (ends with *e*)
pharyng	____________	"throat of the windpipe"
pleur	____________	"rib; side"
cric	____________	"ring"
glott	____________	"tongue"
alveol	____________	"tiny cavity"
ventilat	____________	"fan; blow"
spirat	____________	"breathe"
alkal	____________	"ashes of saltwort" (a base)
acid	____________	"sour"

SINGULAR		PLURAL
bronchus	____________	bronchi
alveolus	____________	alveoli

UNIT 12: SELF-TEST OF WORD PARTS

PREFIXES	MEANING	
par-	____________	"beside"

ROOTS	MEANING	
seros	____________	"serous"
mucos	____________	"mucous"
stalsis	____________	"constriction"

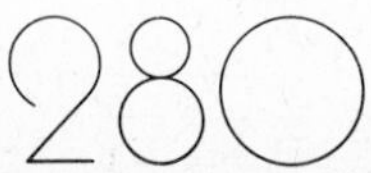

ROOTS	MEANING	
saliv	________	"saliva; spit"
aliment	________	"nourish"
lingu	________	"tongue"
ot	________	"ear"
amyl	________	"starch"
mandibul	________	"little chewer"
prote	________	"protein"
cec	________	"blind"
an	________	"ring"
rug	________	"wrinkle; ditch; furrow"
oment	________	"fat skin"
vill	________	"tuft of hair"
esophag	________	"gullet"
pylor	________	"gatekeeper"
duoden	________	"12 at a time"
jejun	________	"empty; fasting"
ile	________	"flank"
hepat	________	"liver"
splen	________	"spleen"
vermi	________	"worm"
sigm	________	"sigma" (Greek *S*)
intestin	________	"intestine" (ends with *n*)
enter	________	"intestine" (ends with *r*)

SINGULAR		PLURAL
villus	________	villi
ruga	________	rugae

UNIT 13: SELF-TEST OF WORD PARTS

ROOTS	MEANING	
col	__________	"large intestine"
follic	__________	"sac"
glans	__________	"acorn"
clitor	__________	"shut; closed in"
scrot	__________	"bag"
test	__________	"witness; eggshell"
didym	__________	"eggshell"
pen	__________	"tail"
genit	__________	"beget; produce"
trigon	__________	"triangle"
hil	__________	"small trifle"
urin	__________	"urine" (ends with *n*)
urinat	__________	"urine" (ends with *t*)
mictur	__________	"urine" (starts with *m*)
urethr	__________	"urine" (ends with *hr*)
ureter	__________	"urine" (ends with *er*)
juxta	__________	"near"
stat	__________	"stand"
glomerul	__________	"little ball of yarn"
menstru	__________	"month"
uter	__________	"womb" (starts with *u*)
metr	__________	"womb" (starts with *m*)
convolut	__________	"twisted"
corp	__________	"body"

ROOTS	MEANING	
labi	________________	"lip"
semin	________________	"seed; sow"
fund	________________	"base; bottom"
vulv	________________	"wrapper"
vagin	________________	"sheath"
ovulat	________________	"little egg"

SUFFIXES	MEANING	
-ens	________________	"one that"

SINGULAR		PLURAL
calyx	________________	calyces

UNIT 14: SELF-TEST OF WORD PARTS

PREFIXES	MEANING	
ecto-	________________	"outside of"
neo-	________________	"new"

ROOTS	MEANING	
cyst	________________	"bladder"
fet	________________	"offspring"
morul	________________	"little mulberry"
blastul	________________	"little sprouter"
gastrul	________________	"little stomach"
amni	________________	"lamb"
allant	________________	"sausage"

ROOTS	MEANING	
zygot	________	"yoked"
placent	________	"flat cake"
nat	________	"birth; born"

SUFFIXES	MEANING	
-ois	________	"resembling"

INDEX

This is an alphabetical listing of the words, word parts, and abbreviations which appear in blanks within the text. The first set of numbers after each entry refers to the frame number where it is initially used, while the second set of numbers (in **bold type**) indicates the page number of the item.

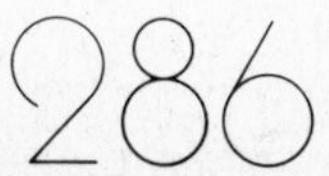

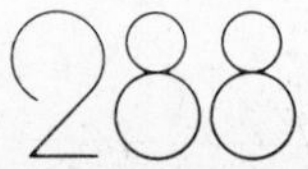

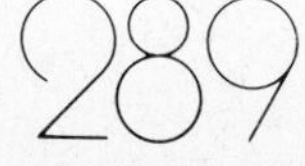

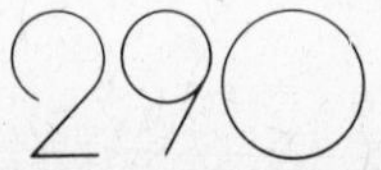

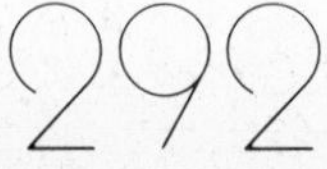